For H and D and S. We grew together.

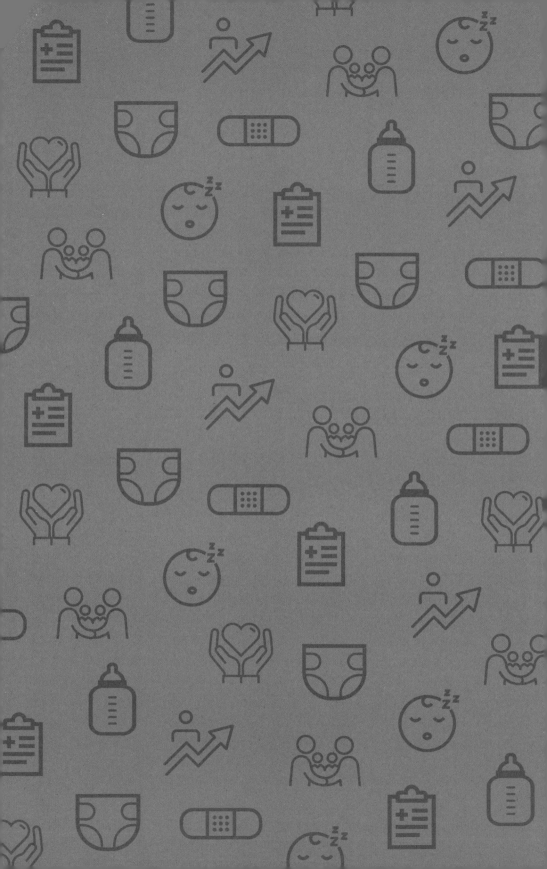

CONTENTS

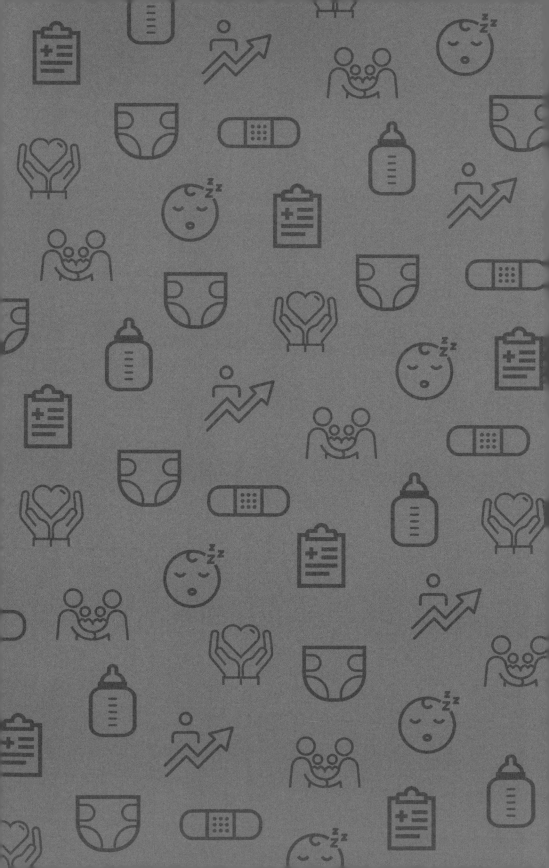

CONGRATS, YOU'RE ABOUT TO BE A NEW DAD!

I'm an experienced father of three grown children and a general pediatrician with over twenty-five years of experience. You'll have a lot to learn on your journey as a dad. You'll do some stuff right and maybe a few things wrong, and that's okay. Perfection is not the goal. You want to raise a good kid, enjoy yourself with your family, and share a few laughs along the way.

Recently, I saw a newborn girl in the office. She was fussing and crying, and her dad was (understandably) a little frustrated. He was holding her and shushing in that way we do with babies, but she was having none of this. I gave him just a little advice—move a little slower, shush a little quieter. Then, I said, try to tell her a joke.

"What joke?"

"Any joke. She just wants to hear you talk. Speak like you're talking to a friend."

In response, he quoted a common "three guys walk into a bar" joke. As he told it, he relaxed. And his baby girl relaxed. And mom relaxed. And soon enough, the room was quiet. Everyone was listening to a guy just being himself and just being a dad.

This book will give you the confidence and knowledge you need to help prepare for and care for your newborn baby from birth through three months. And not just your baby—your job includes helping your partner and taking care of yourself. Kindness, toward your baby, your partner, and yourself, goes a long way.

What you need to know starts right here. It's all based on years of scientific research, my own expertise, and the experiences shared with me from thousands of dads who've made this journey. You can do this, and you can share some jokes along the way.

HOW TO USE THIS BOOK

Things are about to get very busy in your home. You won't have time for a whole lot of reading, so I'm going to leave out the fluff and cover what's most essential.

The first part of this book is about getting ready. We'll talk about the things you need to get and the decisions and discussions that are best done before your baby arrives. We'll cover your baby's birthday—the zeroth birthday, technically—what to expect, what's going to happen, and what you can do to be prepared to help. Then we'll talk about the nuts and bolts of newborn care. There's a lot to do, and you will be ready!

In the second half of the book, we'll focus on your child's needs as they grow from a newborn to a three-month-old baby. There are a great deal of changes in those first few months, and the tricks you'll learn to help a newborn won't work for very long. Never fear. We've got you covered. Feeding, pooping, sleeping, playing—all that good stuff is here.

Throughout the book, I'll use sidebars and short lists to help focus on highlights and issues that are most likely to pop up. You'll also see regular milestone check-ins so you can know your baby is on track. And we'll keep an eye on you, too, Dad—on what you can do to help your partner, your baby, and yourself.

You may want to skim the whole book at once or read relevant sections as you go along. Don't forget to use the index to look for specific concerns as they come up, especially when you're in a hurry. We'll make it easy to find what you need fast. You're ready. Let's go!

Medical Disclaimer: Though I'm a pediatrician, I'm not *your* pediatrician. I don't know the medical particulars about your baby. The information in this book is meant for informational purposes and as a general guide but cannot substitute for specific information from your own medical professional. If you have specific medical questions, ask your doctor.

These icons will help you find big subjects in a hurry (new dads are busy!). The colors also highlight smaller sections if you're looking for more advice on a certain subject.

 Medical: Advice on working with doctors and hospitals, as well as anything that might require you to go visit one.

 Diapering: These sections will give you information on keeping baby fresh and help you understand what you can learn from poop.

 Feeding: What you need to know about keeping your baby eating right and eating often.

 Sleeping: Your baby is going to get a lot of sleep, even if you don't. These sections help you figure out how to build healthy habits.

 Safety: Practical information about protecting your baby from accidental harm.

 Self-Care: These sections have info on navigating the internal struggles you'll face as a new dad.

 Partnership: Highlights sections that offer tips on how to create the strong partnership all parents need.

 Development: Every baby is different, so healthy can mean a lot of things. These sections help you set expectations and offer insight into what's going on.

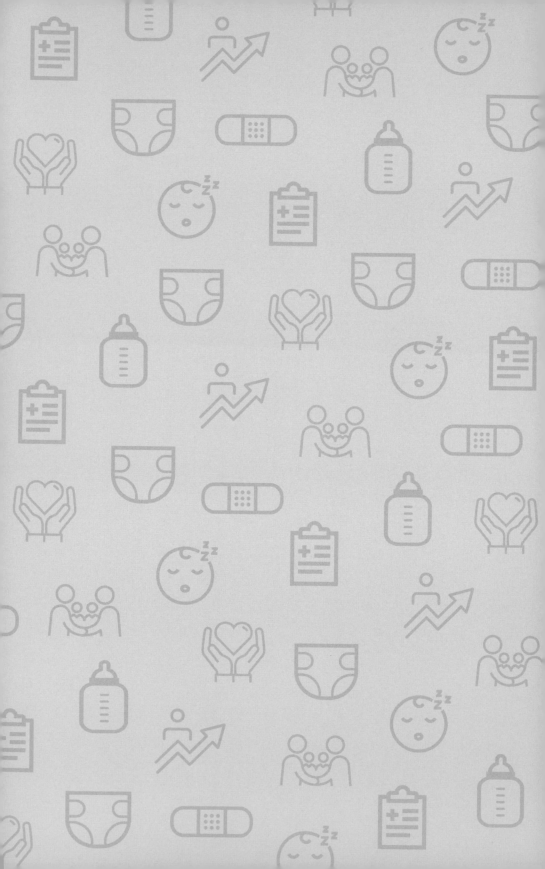

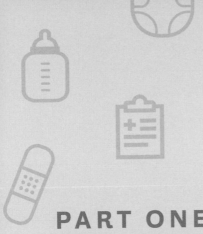

PART ONE

GETTING READY FOR YOUR NEWBORN

CHAPTER ONE

PREPARING FOR FATHERHOOD

Becoming a new dad starts with preparation. There's a lot of things you can do to get ready, and Future Dad will be very thankful that you did the prep work to set the stage for success. In this chapter, we'll start with your mindset. What should you be focusing on, mentally, to be in the right place when the time comes? The Stoic philosopher Seneca said, "We suffer more in imagination than in reality." There's a lot you could worry about, but the reality is there are only a few key things worth your time and attention. They are not complicated, but they're important. Keeping your mind in the right place now will help you and your partner feel more comfortable, more confident, and less worried.

TRUST YOURSELF: YOU'VE GOT THIS

You've known a lot of dads, and you probably already have a mental picture of what you want to become when you're a dad. Trust yourself. You're becoming a dad, yes, but you're still yourself. It's your own life and values that will make you the kind of dad you want to be.

The biggest confidence-killing, doubt-creating pitfall I see is falling into the comparison trap. This may have started already, unintentionally. Try not to compare your partner's pregnancy with others. She may be radiant and happy; she may be tired and grumpy. Maybe she's actively nesting, or maybe she's a couch potato. Some days, she's probably all these things. What's most important is that she's her own person, experiencing her own journey. There's no "wrong" way to be pregnant.

Likewise, when your baby arrives, there will be surprises. Since you'll be new at this, and because the stakes feel so high, you'll be looking for a frame of reference to use. It's a trap! Don't compare yourself or your baby to the others around you. Remember: Different isn't wrong or bad. There are a lot of ways to be a baby and a lot of ways to be a dad. It's great to ask questions and ask for help; you may find new solutions and better ways to do things. That does not mean you (or your partner) were doing something wrong.

READY YOUR RELATIONSHIPS

Everyone is focused on the baby right now, but your relationships with your partner, family, and friends are incredibly important for your physical and emotional health, too. Changes are coming and with them all kinds of new stress and triggers to manage. How you communicate with your partner and with those closest to you can make a lot of difference as you transition together into new identities and new lifestyles. Get into the habit of open, clear communication now to help avoid misunderstandings later.

Parenting is hard work. You'll both be tired and sometimes bad-tempered and sometimes low on the mental and physical energy you'll need to get the job done. A strong, positive relationship with your partner helps both of you be better parents. Having different styles can help both of you better work through problems. Play to each other's strengths, be cooperative and supportive, and keep sharing smiles and positivity along the way.

I'll give you one short, easy exercise to practice even before your baby arrives. To help get in the habit of working together in a positive way, replace the word "but" with the word "and" in your responses. For example:

Partner: "Little Charlie is crying a lot. I'm going to give them some gas drops."

You: "Okay, good idea, but I should turn on the white noise machine."

See what the "but" did there? You acknowledged the good idea, then you kind of sabotaged it by implying it wouldn't work and that you would have to step in. Instead, get used to saying it this way:

You: "Okay, good idea, and I should turn on the white noise machine."

The meaning is completely different. Now you agreed it's a good idea, and you also offered to help! Remember, the word "but" can be a barrier to collaboration and working together; "and" is a way of staying on the same path. Or if you want a quick and childish way to remember this, "but" is for butts.

YOUR FAMILY AND FRIENDS

New parents need all the help they can get. If you're lucky, you have family and friends with a lot of baby experience. Grandparents in particular can be a great resource for sharing newborn work that needs to get done. Even simple things—laundry, shopping, housecleaning—become overwhelming when you're running on four hours of sleep.

The catch is you'll need to actively manage these extra helpers. They mean well but don't always know what to do. It can help to be thankful and explicit at the same time: "Thanks for bringing dinner! Now mom and I really need some quiet time on our own. We'll call you soon." Or even "It's been fun having you here, and I'm glad you got to hold Stephen. Now it's time for his nap so we're going to put him down. Do you have time to help fold some laundry before you go? I'd appreciate it."

You'll also be dealing with unsolicited advice. Remember, you can listen without arguing, and sometimes that's the easiest way. Listen, nod, then ignore. You'll hear from a lot of "experts" on parenting, but you and your partner will always be the experts on your own baby.

YOUR PARENTING APPROACH

There is no one right way to be a parent. Your parenting style is going to be an expression of your own personality. That's great. You will have a more successful and enjoyable time parenting if you act like yourself rather than trying to be someone you're not.

This is true for your partner, too. Having two different parenting styles is a strength. Some challenges will be better tackled by one style than the other. Your skills and strengths can complement each other. Your parenting style will also change and adapt as you grow as a parent. Don't try to be perfect or rigid. Kids are complicated, and different styles will fit different situations. Be kind to yourself and your partner, no matter what kind of parents you're both becoming.

Here's a partial list of some popular parenting styles. Keep in mind that there are many more, and styles can blend together.

INSTINCTIVE PARENTING

Acting on your own instincts, without a lot of advance planning or research, is one common style. Kids raised by instinctive parents can be quick to make decisions and deal with unexpected situations.

AUTHORITATIVE PARENTING

The authority here is you; what you say goes. But there should be some room for flexibility. Children raised by authoritative parents often learn to do things the correct way the first time. Overly authoritative parents may run into more anger and rebellious feelings from their children as they grow.

FREE-RANGE PARENTING

In free-range parenting, the children take charge, with parents following along to (hopefully) keep things safe and moving forward. For young babies, that may mean not stressing over sleep and meal schedules, embracing spontaneity and surprises. Free-range children may become especially independent and self-reliant.

GENTLE PARENTING

Here, parents are in charge and always looking at decisions through the lens of their children's viewpoint. What would they want? What are they expressing? Children raised by gentle parents learn empathy and kindness.

PARENTING CLASSES

Parenting classes can help you feel prepared and reduce your stress. You'll also have a chance to mix with other couples and share one another's experiences. It's a good first step to meeting potential playmates for your child.

Some classes will be focused on specific topics, like infant CPR or labor and birthing. You'll also find courses that cover basic newborn care, strengthening parent relationships, and preparing a safe home for a baby.

Classes are often offered at obstetricians' offices, community centers, libraries, and religious centers. There are both in-person and online options, so pick what works best for you. You can find them on community bulletin boards, social media, and via internet searches. Usually the costs are low, and the investment in time and money is worthwhile.

One caveat: Some parenting classes are geared to sell you products or services. I would stay away from classes sponsored by stores or service providers.

YOUR BIRTH PLAN

A birth plan is a document you both create ahead of time to try to address some of the expectations you'll have about the birth experience. Sometimes they include a lot of details and are developed with a doula or birth coach. Some couples just fill in a brief form, use an online template, or skip a birth plan altogether—any of these options is fine. It's all about making sure the birth parent has a plan everyone is comfortable with following.

Typical choices addressed in a birth plan might include who's on the birth team, what kind of labor mom prefers, pain management, immediate postpartum care, and even things like the mood or vibes in the delivery room. For medical decisions (like circumcision or medical procedures performed on mom or baby before or after birth), please discuss pros and cons with your obstetrician or midwife and your baby's pediatrician. Do what's safest to ensure a healthy mom and baby.

Birth plans are important and a good starting point, but they're just a starting point. Circumstances may lead to unexpected changes, and that's okay.

QUESTIONS TO ASK YOUR OB-GYN

By now, you've probably been working with your partner's obstetrician or midwife for several months. As the delivery date draws near, make sure you both feel comfortable with your knowledge of a few key questions.

- When is your next appointment?
- Are there any other tests or procedures needed, like another ultrasound or follow-up on any previous labs or screening results?
- Is there anything you need to talk with a pediatrician or neonatologist about now?
- What are the signs of labor and preterm labor?
- What should you do or not do during labor?
- What are other reasons to contact the obstetrician's office immediately versus during office hours?
- When should you call the obstetrician during labor, and exactly how do you call?
- What should signal you to drive to the hospital or call 911 immediately?

If you have any plans to vacation or leave town late in pregnancy, be sure to have a backup plan in place.

PREPARING FOR DIFFICULT SITUATIONS

Surprises are bound to happen—sometimes good, sometimes less good. No matter how smoothly pregnancy has gone so far, unpredictable things can come up when a baby is born. In this section, I'll give you a brief overview of some health challenges that may unexpectedly arise for mother or baby as well as some insight into how to manage the stress and anxiety that can accompany them.

PREMATURE BABIES

Human gestation—the length of pregnancy—is forty weeks, or about nine months. But babies are notoriously bad at reading calendars and seldom arrive on their exact due date. Most babies are born between the beginning of the thirty-eighth week and the end of the fortieth week of pregnancy.

A baby born early, before the end of the thirty-seventh week of pregnancy, is called premature. In the United States, that's about 10 percent of births. It's fairly common. You likely know couples who've had babies born premature, and you know adults who were born premature.

If your baby is born early, there may be some extra health challenges or medical steps that will be needed. Trouble tends to focus on breathing and/or eating. Sometimes feeding can start off rocky, or a baby will need an incubator to stay warm. Overall, health problems become more common as babies are born more prematurely. Babies born before thirty-five weeks may have more challenges than babies who almost make it to term; babies born even earlier will need more support. A specialty-trained pediatrician called a neonatologist who works at the hospital, will lead your premature baby's medical team if necessary.

Babies who are born prematurely may seem to lag developmentally compared with babies of the same age who were born at term. But don't worry. If you "correct" their age by accounting for the prematurity, development should be right on track. For instance, if your baby is born two months early, subtract two months from their age when looking at developmental milestones. When your baby is four months old, they'll have reached the developmental stage of a two-month-old; at six months of age, they'll be at four-month milestones. They catch up but need time to grow, learn, and mature.

WHAT ELSE TO LOOK OUT FOR

Here's a brief, partial list of some other more common medical issues that come up after birth. You'll learn more about these from your physicians if you need to.

Breech: Most babies develop in a head-down position or at least move to that position before the end of pregnancy. A baby who stays sideways—or "breech"—may have a more difficult delivery.

Failure to progress: I don't like this term, but we're stuck with it. When a baby isn't moving down the birth canal to make their way out, it's called "failure to progress." Medicine can help, or sometimes a C-section is needed.

Preeclampsia: This can be a complication during pregnancy, causing high blood pressure and serious health problems for mom and baby. Sometimes an early delivery will be needed to protect everyone's health.

Jaundice: All newborns turn just a little yellowish, but if it's more than a little, there can be problems. A blood test called a "bilirubin" will be used to measure the amount of jaundice. If it's too elevated, treatment may be needed to prevent any lasting problems.

Heart murmur: This is a kind of noise from the heart, and it's very common in newborns. Most murmurs are not a problem and can be monitored by your nurses and pediatrician; some will require additional testing or a specialist's input.

Birth injuries: Giving birth can be difficult, and injuries can occur to mom or baby. The most common baby birth injuries are bruises. More rarely, there can be fractures of bones or nerve damage. All of these usually heal well. You'll have your pediatrician's guidance on what to look for and what, if anything, needs to be done.

LIFE IN THE NICU

If your baby is more than a few weeks premature or has significant health problems, they'll probably receive care in a neonatal intensive care unit (NICU). This is the absolute best place for these babies to be, but it can be scary or overwhelming for families.

The first thing you'll notice is that NICUs are dark and quiet. Premature babies don't like a lot of loud sounds and bright lights. NICU babies usually live in a covered incubator to keep warm or a raised bed with a gentle warmer overhead. Some babies may be hooked up to monitors and breathing equipment.

Like other ICUs, NICUs will have rules about who can visit and when. That's to keep noise down and prevent infections. At first, there may be a rush to do a lot of medical things, but once your baby is settled, you'll be encouraged to visit. Your baby wants you to come and wants you to hold them when you can.

Your NICU team will stay in touch to help you help your baby best. You may also want to get involved with parent support groups, especially if your baby will need more than a brief NICU stay. Your NICU staff will have a list of local resources to share. You (and your baby) are not alone.

COPING WITH STRESS

People facing difficult and unexpected situations can feel stressed and overwhelmed. You or your partner may have obsessive thoughts, extreme worry, or panic attacks. Remember that your reaction isn't abnormal or weird. The nurses and doctors taking care of your baby have helped many parents through difficult times. Lean on them for their help, and share how you feel. Encourage your partner to do the same. The important thing to remember is that all that expensive equipment, all that cutting-edge science, and all those highly trained people are focused on your baby's health. Similar to saying "and" instead of "but," this is an exercise in perspective. You don't "have" to be in the NICU; you "should" be. Positivity and gratitude will get you through it more easily than fear and self-pity.

Other steps that help some people cope with stress include the following:

- Getting out of the hospital, at least for a little while
- Do what you would normally do, such as a sport or hobby
- Exercising
- Talking to supportive friends and family

If you feel your or your partner's worries are unmanageable, please talk to your hospital care team and your own physician. Postpartum depression is always a concern and should be part of health screenings your partner has after the baby has been born. For more info on postpartum depression, see page 62.

HOW TO SUPPORT YOUR PARTNER

Everyone copes with difficult medical situations differently, and you and your partner can help each other through this. Sometimes that means just listening to each other; sometimes it helps to trouble-shoot and come up with solutions; and sometimes it's best to offer a quiet and supportive hug. (Be gentle. Mom just had a baby!) Little things like getting her preferred clothing, shampoo, and toothpaste can go a long way, too. Be there both mentally and physically, and you'll be helping.

It can also help to focus on the little things that you can control. Try to make sure your partner is eating well or at least as well as she can in a hospital (go get takeout if necessary). Protect her sleep. Help her stay focused on the decisions you need to make now, rather than worrying about what might happen next.

CHAPTER TWO

SUPPORT, SAFETY, AND THE ESSENTIALS

t's nuts and bolts time! In this chapter, we're going to focus on the essential things you need to do before your baby arrives. You'll need to pick a doctor, plan for childcare, and get your home safe and ready. You'll also want to make a plan for contacting family and friends and for handling visitors and neighbors. There are tons of things you *can* buy—those lists from the baby store are enormous!—but do you need all that stuff right now? Short answer: no. Long answer: read on!

CHOOSING A PEDIATRICIAN

Your newborn will have their own doctor, a specialist in the care of children. This will usually be a pediatrician, who should be "board certified" by the American Board of Pediatrics. Most of us are also members or "fellows" of the American Academy of Pediatrics (AAP), so we'll have some extra initials in our title: Roy Benaroch, MD, FAAP. That's not a guarantee of a good doc, but it's a good start.

Some families work with "family practice" physicians, who receive broader training in taking care of both children and adults. They won't have quite the depth of experience with children, especially with babies who are sick or have special needs or kids with complex diagnoses. You may also find a physician marked as a DO instead of an MD. These are the names of the two medical degrees offered by American medical schools: doctor of osteopathy and doctor of medicine. Functionally, the training is essentially the same, and as long as they completed a pediatric residency training and are board certified, either is fine.

Beyond the basic qualifications, what's most important is finding a physician who's up-to-date on pediatric care, listens well, and fits your style of parenting. Some parents prefer a very direct, "just tell me exactly what I need to know" kind of doc. Other parents feel more comfortable with someone who'll discuss and troubleshoot and work more collaboratively to find solutions. Some pediatricians like to play and laugh along with parents; other parents prefer a doctor who's going to stay more serious and focused.

You may also have preferences about the age and gender of your doc or how long they've been in practice. Visiting with prospective pediatricians during prenatal visits can help you get some insights. You can also network on social media and ask neighbors about their experiences.

There are practical considerations, too. Is the practice "in network" with your insurance or Medicaid program? Are they close enough for you to get to the office quickly if something unexpected comes up? Is parking easy? Is it a bigger, dynamic practice with a lot of providers or a smaller practice with fewer doctors? How's their after-hours access? Do they have a portal for messages and paperwork like day care intake forms?

It's best to pick your practice and doctor in advance and maybe even a backup, too. But keep in mind that you may not find a pediatric practice that fulfills everything you're looking for. You may be constrained by geography or insurance. Many families have to prioritize what's most important to make a first or second choice. Don't stress over perfection here. You'll realize after your baby is born that some of your priorities will have changed anyway. If you don't mesh or connect well or you realize you need something different, you can change pediatricians after a baby is born. There's no penalty. What's most important is that you find a comfortable medical home that fits your needs in the long run.

PLANNING FOR CHILDCARE

Many families feel a bit overwhelmed thinking in advance about childcare, but it's important. You're going to need at least some help taking care of your baby, and you'll have more and better options if you make decisions and get the legwork done early. Talk with your partner about your combined needs: how you'll work around timing drop-offs and pickups and the costs of each option. These are just some of the many decisions that are best made together.

BABYSITTERS

A babysitter traditionally provides short-term care for a baby or child and usually lacks formal training. Care can take place at your home or at the sitter's home and might involve just your baby or just one or two more children, sometimes of varying ages (you should know exactly what to expect in advance, of course). These days, informal sitters in neighborhoods provide a lot of care. Sometimes they are older women who've raised their own kids or younger women who are part-time workers or students. There's often flexibility in hours, though the trade-off is you'll have to work around their schedule, too, and there will be no easy or automatic backup plan. Networking to find a sitter typically begins with neighbors or at local churches, synagogues, or schools. Ask for references, and make calls to vet recommendations. Even if you choose one of the more formal options below as your main childcare, it's great to have a few sitters lined up for unexpected or off-hours needs.

A NANNY OR AN AU PAIR

A nanny is an experienced professional; their full-time job is to take care of children. Though they'll often have extensive experience and sometimes formal training, there are few regulations, and you'll have to ask about qualifications and check references carefully. You'll also want to talk about your parenting style and expectations. Nannies can be a little set in their ways, and disagreements about childcare decisions can come up.

An au pair is a young adult, most often a woman, who's from a foreign country. She'll come to live in your home for up to a few years. In exchange for providing full-time childcare, you'll house and feed her and provide a stipend. Having an au pair can be an affordable option, but you'll need to screen carefully. Think about your home and privacy and if you wish to have someone live with you long term. Bonus: Your baby may have a unique chance to learn a second language.

If you choose an au pair or nanny, remember to also develop a backup plan if your caretaker becomes ill or has an emergency.

DAY CARE CENTERS

Day care centers can be more affordable than one-on-one care from a nanny, and you know they'll stay open and available with reliable hours. There are often wait lists, so you need to line up a day care center in advance. You'll want a place that's fully licensed and insured and hires well-qualified people, preferably fully vaccinated.

Try to choose a location that's close to home and work so it's easier to drop off and pick up (including inevitable days when your baby gets sick during the day). Make sure to look at the ratio of staff to babies. When choosing, make multiple advance visits, and pop in at unexpected times. Some things to consider include these questions: Is the staff happy? Do they seem stressed and preoccupied? How clean is the facility? (Don't expect perfection. A certain amount of clutter is fine.) Bigger day cares will have multiple "rooms," dedicated by age groups, which is typically safer and limits infections. Whatever day care you choose, plan on your child getting at least a few extra colds and tummy bugs, especially their first year. Even the cleanest, most careful day care centers become a source of infections for babies and their parents.

FRIENDS AND FAMILY

Friend and family childcare can be a great option, but you have to be realistic about your expectations. Friends cannot be expected to regularly work for free. If you're lucky and have a friend (or two!) who also has childcare needs, you may be able to work out a rotation to share the load, trading off by days or weeks. The logistics may be tricky and may require some workplace flexibility, but it's a good solution if you can put it together.

Having family available for routine care can be wonderful for everyone. But again, you have to be honest and realistic. Not all grandparents want to be full-time sitters, and not all grandparents are physically capable. You may also need to set up boundaries to ensure that you, the parent, remain the "decider." In the past, multigenerational families sharing a house or home meant built-in day care and a job for every generation, and I think that can still be a great alternative. As always, communication and honesty are needed to make sure this kind of collaborative relationship is best for your family.

WORKING FROM HOME

In the postpandemic era, it has become increasingly common for one (or both) parents to obtain a remote work position that allows them to stay home and care for their child as well as earn a steady paycheck. The advantages are obvious. Who better to care for your child than you? And sidestepping a hefty day care bill makes great economic sense. But many parents don't see the long-term challenges. Caring for a baby at home is work; you will not be able to concentrate 100 percent on your day job. Balancing employer expectations and baby needs can be difficult. As your baby grows, they'll need different kinds of attention. There's also a high risk of burnout for parents who never get to feel "off the clock" from either responsibility. You should develop a routine that incorporates out-of-the-house breaks and assigns chores in advance to help avoid this.

VISITORS AND YOUR NEWBORN

There isn't a one-size-fits-all approach to visitors during the newborn period. You should think of decisions about visitors as a balance: Yes, visitors may be more likely to expose your child to infections, and those can hit newborns harder. But you will need some help, and especially close family members will be eager to meet your baby. Bottom line: Do what's best for your baby and your family.

To minimize the downside, try to limit visits to your closest family and friends. Ask people who may be sick to stay home. Everyone who visits should wash their hands. Masking can also prevent the spread of respiratory viruses, but honestly, if anyone has symptoms of a respiratory infection, they shouldn't come visit at all. Toddlers and younger school-age children are the most likely people to carry around infections; you really want to limit visits from young cousins and neighbors, at least for the first few months. Be explicit with your neighbors about the limits you've settled on. I'll also give you permission to blame your baby's doctor. You can say, "We'd love to have you over, but our pediatrician is very strict and made us promise to limit visitors for now."

Visits can have big benefits, too. Encourage helpful visitors to chip in by making dinner, taking care of housework, or holding the baby while you or your partner sleeps. A little chitchat is nice, but what you really need now is someone to tackle the laundry and get things done so you can take a break.

PREPARING YOUR HOME

Your newborn baby will be entirely dependent on you and your partner to keep them safe. It's not super difficult, at least not yet (they're not going to walk around and explore for a while!). Still, there are some things you need to think about.

CREATING A SAFE SLEEP SPACE

For safety, the AAP recommends that the baby sleeps in the same room as their parents, on their own surface separate from their parents' bed, and always put down flat on their backs. Babies should be moved to their own room for night sleep between six to twelve months, depending on parent preference. There are a few essential items you need, some optional items, and a few things you should avoid:

Crib or bassinet (essential): Your baby's crib or bassinet should meet all safety regulations. It's best to buy a new one or a gently used one from a trusted source. Stay away from yard sales for this item; you won't know if it's safe. A crib should be solid, without drop sides, and placed away from windows, heaters, electric and shade cords, and wall decorations. Younger babies can use a smaller, more portable device, sometimes on wheels that can lock. Either way, the sides should be either open between slats or breathable mesh.

Firm mattress (essential): Buy a new mattress, one that fits snugly into your crib or bassinet. It should be firm, with no space or gaps around it, hypoallergenic, and free from toxins like lead and mercury. You'll also need fitted sheets that are nice and snug. Don't use any other bedding—no comforter, no pillows, no soft anything else in the sleeping space. You can find a summary of current crib and mattress safety guidelines on the United States Consumer Product Safety Commission website.

Baby monitor (optional): While not absolutely necessary, many families rely on a good baby monitor that allows you to hear and see your baby, even in the dark. Double-check secure setups for any Wi-Fi-enabled devices as these can be easily hacked if you aren't careful.

Swaddler (optional): Many young babies seem to sleep better in a good swaddle. You can learn to make one with a receiving blanket (ask one of the nurses at the hospital), or you can use a special blanket, often with Velcro, to make it easy. If you're the type that struggles folding laundry, it can be a great investment. Stop using these products around two months or when your baby is starting to try to roll over.

Inclined sleepers (avoid): Sleepers that position babies at an inclined angle have been recalled and banned because they've caused infant deaths. If you see one at a garage sale, tell the owner to destroy it. Do not use inclined sleepers.

Sleep positioners (avoid): We know it's safest to put a baby down to sleep on their back. But you don't want to use anything that *keeps* them on their back. Straps, wedges, and the like are dangerous.

CREATING A SAFE CHANGING SPACE

You and your partner will be changing a lot of diapers. You need a safe and comfortable place to do this, a place where your baby can't roll away and where you can comfortably reach everything you need while keeping one hand on them. You will also need the following:

- **Diapers:** You'll go through a lot of them, but don't buy too many just at first. You don't know how big your baby will be or how fast they'll outgrow the newborn size.

- **Baby wipes:** Commercial baby wipes are gentle and convenient. These days, they're usually unscented and free of alcohol and harsh chemicals. Just don't flush them down the toilet.

- **A sturdy table:** Get one that's easy to clean and has a comfortable and washable topper or pad. Make sure the height is good for you and your partner to use without too much bending.

- **A good bin:** There are clever gizmos that package up disposable diapers each in their own plastic sleeve to minimize odors and keep things tidy.

- **A place for laundry:** Changing diapers is a little messy sometimes. Even experts occasionally end up needing to change a baby's clothes, too. Keep clean clothes and a place for dirty clothes nearby.

- **Diaper rash cream:** No matter how often you change your baby, an occasional rash is going to appear. Dry well, then leave the bottom naked for a while. Then you'll want to use a low-cost diaper cream that contains about 20 percent zinc oxide. The more expensive products do not work any better.

BABYPROOFING FOR NEWBORNS

Babyproofing means keeping your home safe for your baby. The exact steps you'll need will depend to some degree on their developmental stage. Once they start crawling, for instance, you need to make sure they can't get to the stairs. For now, you'll want to concentrate on the immediate things necessary for a safe home for a newborn and also for the adults who will be carrying them around.

- Set your hot water heater to 120 degrees Fahrenheit or less.

- Install smoke alarms with fresh batteries on every floor of your home.

- If you have gas appliances or an attached garage, install carbon monoxide detectors, too.

- Install fire extinguishers, especially in kitchens and laundry/utility rooms, and make sure you know how to use them.

- Fix peeling or flaking paint. If your home was built before 1978, it could contain lead. Find professionals to test and deal with it.

- Put nonslip pads under rugs and nonslip strips on stairs.

- Get in the habit of unplugging and storing electrical appliances that aren't in use, especially clothes irons and curling irons.

- Make sure cords from blinds and curtains can be tucked away with secure cord stops. Or get rid of all dangling cords entirely.

VOLATILE ORGANIC COMPOUNDS

Volatile organic compounds (VOCs) are man-made chemicals found in cleaners, solvents, paints, and fuels. They are emitted as gases, often with strong odors, and are dangerous in closed indoor spaces. Because babies breathe more rapidly and have a higher lung surface area proportionally than adults, they are more susceptible to health problems from these chemicals. VOCs can cause breathing problems (both short- and long-term) and have been linked to an increased risk of chronic illnesses like cancer.

To limit your newborn's exposures to VOCs, do any home renovating at least eight weeks before your baby's expected arrival. This includes stripping, painting, and wallpapering. If you use these kinds of chemicals as a hobby or in your work, set aside a separate area to change clothes well away from your baby. If you must use these chemicals in your home with a baby, keep windows open to increase ventilation as much as possible. Air purifiers with activated carbon filters can help. As a general rule, if you can smell the chemicals, then they are a danger to your baby, as your baby's exposure is much higher than yours.

YOUR NEWBORN'S MUST-HAVE ITEMS

We've talked about sleep and diaper changes and the supplies you'll need for safety and convenience. But you're not done shopping yet. Just a few more things will round out your "must-have" list.

CAR SEAT

You can't take your baby home from the hospital without a safe, age-appropriate car seat. Buy it new. Car seats that are older or ones that have already been in an accident are no longer reliable and should never be sold or reused. Car seats sold at major retailers will all meet safety standards and will be rear-facing, as required by law. Many of them can be clicked into a base that stays fixed in your car and can also click safely into a stroller device. Pretty slick. Make sure to install it correctly in your vehicle, ideally in the middle of a middle row or back seat. If you're not sure how to choose or install a car seat, refer to the United States Department of Transportation's National Highway Traffic Safety Administration (NHTSA) website dedicated to car seats and booster seats. Police and fire stations can also provide assistance.

FEEDING SUPPLIES

If mom is planning to nurse exclusively, you may not end up needing much in the way of feeding supplies, just a few burp cloths. Some nursing moms will also use a breast pump; most insurance plans will cover these. It wouldn't be a bad idea to have a basic kit for bottle-feeding: just a few empty bottles and some formula powder or premixed, ready-to-feed formula to use if you end up in a pinch.

For families who'll be bottle-feeding or blended feeding, you'll want a dozen or so bottles and nipples, cleaning brushes, and infant formula (which is usually in powdered form, the most economical and easiest to store). You may need to experiment with different bottle and nipple styles to find what seems most comfortable for your baby. The more expensive or "premium" bottles aren't always better. A bottle drying rack can be handy to keep things organized.

BATHING SUPPLIES

Get a tub insert for your kitchen sink. You'll be able to stand comfortably during bath time, using the sink sprayer or faucet. You'll also want some small, soft washcloths, baby soap, baby shampoo, and a hooded towel with bunny or puppy ears sewn in. (Okay, that's less essential but adorable. Have fun!)

OTHER BABY CARE

The last few essentials, I promise! You'll need the following:

- **A diaper bag or backpack:** Something to take when you leave the house.

- **Pacifiers:** Not essential for everyone. If you really don't like these, you don't need them. But for many babies, they're great for helping to soothe and settle.

- **Nursery glider or rocker:** A comfortable place to nurse or bottle-feed.

- **Receiving blankets:** These are for holding babies, laying out a clean surface, or cleaning spit-up in a pinch. Trust me, you want some of these in the home.

- **Clothes:** You probably want more than you think your baby needs. You will need a lot of spare clothes. Don't forget something cozy to sleep in, like a sleep sack.

- **Stroller:** It doesn't have to be super expensive or fancy, but it should be solid and well-made.

- **Basic first aid kit:** Be sure to include a rectal thermometer, adhesive bandages, and antibiotic ointment.

- **Nail clippers and an emery board.** Those little nails get sharp!
- **Laundry detergent:** Verify that it is unscented and hypoallergenic.

SAVING MONEY ON BABY PRODUCTS

Premium prices often don't get you anything better, so don't be fooled by marketing or upscale claims at expensive stores. Since many baby items are used for only a few months, you can often reuse donated or shared baby products, which keeps them out of landfills. Here are some budget-friendly ideas:

- Network with other families with young children. As their babies grow, they'll have things they no longer need; you can swap back and forth. Social media can be a great resource for finding groups in your area that facilitate this.

- Get in touch with your local BuyNothing.org group. These are nonprofit, loosely organized neighborhood groups for giving away and getting gently used household items of all kinds.

- Contact local organizations like religious schools and community associations such as the Moms Helping Moms Foundation, Mother to Mother, and Basics4Babies.

- For families in need, diapers and supplies can be acquired from the National Diaper Bank Network, state Medicaid programs, or directly from diaper manufacturers.

I'd also encourage you to support these organizations when your baby outgrows diapers or other supplies. Donate and help other families.

CHAPTER THREE

THE BIRTH OF YOUR NEWBORN

The big day is here! Usually, you can't schedule this in advance. If your baby is feeling cooperative, birth might occur within a few days of the due date. Or maybe not. Guess what? This won't be the last time you'll have to wing it, Dad. In this chapter, we'll cover your baby's birth and what to expect on that first day, even if it's unexpected.

BIRTH

Your partner is having regular contractions, and you've headed to the hospital or birthing center. You're probably in a private room in an area called labor and delivery, with nurses and techs stopping in to check on you. Your obstetrician or midwife is standing by and may have visited. Sometimes, monitors are placed on mom and maybe on your baby, too, to track vital signs and progress.

Once your baby's head has started to make its way down and the cervix is fully dilated, your birthing team will encourage mom to push. This part can be noisy, quiet, frantic, calm, or anywhere in between. Someone will be down between mom's legs to catch the baby (maybe you've talked about it, and you'll do that part!). First the head comes out, then in one more push, the rest of your baby.

Magic.

Sometimes newborns will begin to cry upon delivery, or sometimes they need a little stimulation to get going. Then, they'll be dried off and checked over quickly. It's time for you and mom to meet your baby!

There's also a chance your partner may need to have a C-section to surgically remove the baby. This is usually a quick procedure compared to potential hours of labor. Either way, once the baby has arrived, here's what happens next.

BABY'S FIRST MOMENTS AND PROCEDURES

A lot goes on in those first moments after your baby is born. The medical team will be focused on the immediate health of the baby, and if they feel any special steps are needed, they'll get started right away. This might mean suctioning mucus, giving some stimulation, or getting your baby dried and under a warmer. There might also be specific parts of the birth plan you and your partner want them to follow, and you may need to speak up. But always, the health of your baby is going to be everyone's priority. Check in with your partner while all this is going on. She's going to want your support.

WHAT YOUR NEWBORN MAY LOOK LIKE

I've seen and held a lot of newborn babies, and I can say this with certainty: They're adorable. And sometimes, they're kind of funny-looking. Here are some normal things you might see. If anything seems unusual or concerning to you, please bring it up with the delivery team and your pediatrician. We've seen it before, and we're happy to explain.

- **Coneheads:** It isn't easy to be born. Sometimes heads get squeezed. That's okay. However, since the bones of the skull haven't fused together yet, they can slide around and overlap. As a result, sometimes heads look kind of misshapen, like a cone. No worries. All will be well in just a few days.

- **Bruising and swelling:** Again, tight squeeze. Your partner and your baby may look bruised and swollen. They'll be fine. Your birth team will know if any special steps are needed for further monitoring.

- **Vernix:** Many newborn babies are covered with a white, creamy film called vernix. It's there to protect the skin. The World Health Organization recommends leaving the vernix in place and waiting at least six hours before the first bath, though many birthing centers in the United States prefer to give baby their first bath earlier to reduce the risk of infection. There's no strong evidence that either approach is best.

SKIN-TO-SKIN CONTACT

After a brief evaluation, your baby will likely be placed in skin-to-skin contact with mom—bare baby, mom's bare chest, under a soft blanket—just to relax. This helps baby settle and get used to the world and helps mom by encouraging the release of hormones that give happy feelings, decrease pain, and help milk come in. If mom wants, she can peek at her baby, sing, or explore with her hands, and you can do these things, too. After a little while, mom can try to nurse for the first time.

Though it's great to have this time together, sometimes medical issues with mom or baby need to be addressed first. Skin-to-skin contact is not essential, and if you miss out on this time, there will be plenty of time for close bonding later. Let the medical team do what they need to do to keep mom and baby safe.

Skin-to-skin contact isn't just for the period immediately after birth. Continue these peaceful, connecting times once you get home, and, Dad, you should do it, too.

FIRST FEEDINGS

Newborns should try to have their first meal soon after birth, usually within an hour and often sooner. The key word here is "try." Sometimes newborns are kind of stunned, sleepy, or just not ready to take that first breast or bottle. Don't get discouraged if your baby is still trying to catch their breath. Your birth team will help with these initial feedings, too.

For the first day or two, most babies need very little intake. They rely on a special kind of stored energy called brown fat to keep their temperature stable and give them a metabolic boost. You should try to feed your baby at least every two to three hours. The volume of each feed may be very low, less than an ounce each time. Your baby may tire quickly at the breast or bottle and fall asleep. That's fine this first day. Your team will keep an eye on things and make sure all is well.

WEIGHT AND MEASUREMENTS

At the birth hospital, the staff will periodically check your baby for several measurements. Vital signs, including temperature, pulse, and respiratory rate, will be checked several times a day. Your baby's length and head circumference will be checked once or twice, and the weight will be checked daily. If any of these numbers raises concern, your team will discuss it with you. If you have questions about any of these, now's the time to ask.

Parents and pediatricians often focus the most attention on weight. All newborns lose weight for the first few days of life, and that's expected and normal because of fluid losses and the metabolism of brown fat. Up to 7 to 10 percent of birth weight may be lost, and that's not concerning. Weight usually bottoms out by day four, and most babies are back to birth weight by the time you visit your pediatrician for a two-week wellness check.

MEDICAL PROCEDURES

Most babies are born healthy. To help keep them healthy, there are several essential medical procedures that will take place in the minutes and hours after birth.

Apgar test, or just "Apgars": Named after its inventor, physician and pediatric hero Virginia Apgar, the Apgar score is a number from zero to ten that reflects the overall health of your baby in the few minutes after birth. The higher and closer to ten, the better, but it isn't a contest. Don't worry if your baby doesn't get a ten. Traditionally, that score only goes to the newborns of pediatricians and labor nurses.

Cord clamping: Once baby is born, they no longer depend on blood from the umbilical cord to bring oxygen from mom's lungs. It's time to breathe on their own! Clamping and then cutting the cord is the first step toward physiological independence. Dad, if you want to do this step yourself, talk with the birth team beforehand.

Eye drops: The United States Preventive Services Task Force, the American Academy of Pediatrics, and organizations all over the globe recommend antibiotic eye ointment to prevent infections in all newborns. It's simple, safe, and effective.

Vitamin K injection: In the past, some babies developed serious bleeding in their brains or intestines after birth, with devastating consequences. A quick, safe injection of vitamin K eliminates the risk. All babies should get this.

Hepatitis B vaccine: To prevent neonatal transmission of hepatitis B, one vaccine is given in the days after birth. It's safe, effective, and recommended worldwide.

Newborn screening: All U.S. states have mandatory screening in place for serious, treatable metabolic conditions, hearing loss, and heart disease. These tests are inexpensive, and a negative test is super reassuring. A positive or abnormal screening doesn't mean there's a definite problem, but it does mean additional testing will be needed.

Some optional things: Depending on circumstances, your baby may have some additional tests, like checking blood sugar or measuring jaundice. Rely on your care team and pediatrician to explain why these are needed and what they mean.

COMMON CONDITIONS AFTER BIRTH

There are many common medical conditions that can occur shortly after birth. Most of these are essentially normal or very low risk, but it can help your anxiety to know what to expect.

- **Newborn rashes:** Newborn skin undergoes a huge change from inside (always the same temperature, always underwater) to outside, and there are a whole lot of different rashes that newborns get. Most are normal, including red splotches, little whiteheads, and acne-looking spots. Ask about any rashes that concern you. The only newborn rash that may be of some medical urgency is a rash that looks like little blisters. Bring that to a nurse's attention as it could be a sign of neonatal herpes, a very serious infection.

- **Jaundice:** Almost all babies turn at least a little yellow in the days after birth. Your team can measure this with a test called a "bilirubin." Sometimes, an overly high bilirubin is treated with special lights or extra fluids.

- **Purple hands and feet:** Technically called acrocyanosis, this is a normal finding in newborns and young babies. They're not low in oxygen. It's caused by immature circulation and is not a problem.

- **Vaginal discharge:** Female babies can have a milky or bloody vaginal discharge at first, and it's normal.

CIRCUMCISION DECISION

Many male newborns in the United States undergo circumcision, which is the surgical removal of the tubular skin at the end of the penis (the foreskin). Some families request circumcision for cultural, religious, or other personal reasons. Other families prefer to leave the foreskin intact.

There are some small medical advantages of circumcision: Your baby will have a lower risk of urinary tract infections and, later in life, a reduced risk of penis cancer. However, these risks are very small to begin with. Weighing against circumcision are some disadvantages, too, primarily the small risk of a botched procedure.

This is a decision that parents should make, informed by input from their pediatrician and obstetrician. Either way, almost all families (and boys) are happy with how things turn out.

CHAPTER FOUR

BASIC NEWBORN CARE

N ewborns are sturdier than you think. Hold them. Play with them. They will not break. Of course, they do need some special attention and care. They grow fast, but they'll be counting on their families for every-thing they need to thrive and stay safe. You can be a big part of this. It's time to talk about how to hold and dress a newborn and how to help keep them clean and happy. A lot of your focus will be on feeding, pooping, and sleeping, so we'll cover those topics, too. Let's dive in!

BUILDING AND KEEPING A SCHEDULE

You and your partner are probably used to having a basic schedule to your lives. You more or less eat at around the same times, sleep on a schedule, and do what you need to do when you need to do it. With a newborn in your home, all this will change. Your baby can't tell time. They have no idea if it's time for morning coffee or Monday Night Football.

For the first days or weeks, it really is better to follow your baby's lead. Feed when they're hungry, let them sleep when they want to sleep, and hold and play with them when they're awake. Even in those first few weeks, though, pay attention to patterns, and look out for any routines starting to develop. Once your baby starts to fall into a rhythm, reinforce it by aiming to do things at the times when they "usually" want to.

You won't be able to enforce schedules rigidly, but you'll see that over time a typical schedule will emerge that you can build on. There will be some ups and downs, but you will regain control of your day, and you'll even be able to count on quiet time with your partner again. Soon.

HOLDING AND SUPPORT

Newborns have relatively large and heavy heads, and they lack the strong neck muscles needed to hold their heads up on their own. When you pick up a newborn, use one hand behind their head, over their neck, for support. Your other hand can scoop behind the back or buttocks. You don't need to rigidly hold or squeeze the head— some motion is just fine—but provide support to prevent the head from falling back toward the floor and stretching in an uncomfortable way.

Babies like to be held, and there are several different ways to do it. You'll find a position that's comfortable and cozy for both of you. You can cradle your baby across one arm, with their head near your shoulder and your hand supporting their bottom; that's a great way to see your baby's face and talk to them. Or you can hold a baby with their face looking over your shoulder, patting their back or bottom for comfort. Another good hold is a one-handed, running-back football hold, with the face or the back of their head in your hand and their body supported by your forearm (baby can face up or down). This keeps your other hand free for a TV remote or your eleventh cup of coffee.

The important thing here is that you feel confident and comfortable and happy holding your baby. Believe me, your baby wants you to hold them. That skin-to-skin contact is reassuring for both of you. You'll find a hold that you both like and one that feels secure and safe.

Speaking of safety: Don't carry a hot drink or anything sharp along with your baby. Be careful on stairs, too, especially if you're tired, and turn on some lights at night if you're walking around.

CLOTHES AND DRESSING

You may want some frillier or more hip clothes for photos, but most of the time you'll want your newborn dressed in simple, soft clothes that are comfortable and easy to change and wash.

You won't find a lot of zippers on newborn clothes, since they can pinch skin. Buttons? A hassle. Instead, get used to little metal or plastic snaps. Often, there will be extra snaps and flaps to make a larger opening to help get that big newborn head in and out. For outfits with snaps all down the legs, it's easier to get things started if you snap one or two at the bottom before you put it on. Trying to align a half dozen snaps on a wiggling, fussy baby in the dead of night is as frustrating as it sounds.

Some babies really don't like to be changed. Try to make this step easier by talking and singing while looking at your baby's face. Reassure your baby (and yourself!) that all will be well as soon as you get these socks back on.

HYGIENE

Good skin care and hygiene will help keep your newborn comfortable and healthy, and bonus, you'll enjoy that "new baby" scent!

BATHING AND SKIN CARE

Newborns don't get super dirty, but they do need a bath now and then. If your baby finds bath time relaxing and enjoyable, feel free to bathe every day. If your baby hates it, twice a week is probably fine. Babies who are a little more spitty might need to be bathed more often or at least get a touch-up and a change of clothes. Ordinary, in-a-tub baths can start once the umbilical cord falls off. Until then, avoid submerging your baby in water and just do sponge baths, one section at a time.

Most important: Keep baby safe during bath time. Your hot water heater should be set at no higher than 120 degrees Fahrenheit (50 degrees Celsius), and you should always test the water temperature with your hand. You can use a regular bathroom tub, but it's much easier at first to bathe them in the kitchen sink using a tub insert. Always keep one hand on your baby while they're in the tub, and don't walk away even for a second. Make sure everything you need is in reach before you start, and call for help if you need something else. If you must interrupt bath time and no one else can take over, take your baby out of the water.

The bath time order should look like this: prep the water (plain water, no soap yet), then get your baby naked, then into the tub. Enjoy some splashy time with the plain water if you'd like. Then use a little baby soap on a small soft washcloth, first face, then neck (don't forget the neck folds), then arms, legs, body, back, and last the diaper area. You won't need to scrub, and honestly you can probably skip the soap on the face, at least sometimes. Afterward, a gentle dry off, followed by moisturizing cream if you'd like. The whole time, stay safe by keeping a hand on baby.

DIAPER CARE

Newborn skin is a little less waterproof and a little more sensitive, so frequent diaper changes are a good idea. Definitely change as soon as possible if there's any poop, and change wet diapers when it's practical (don't wake a baby to change a diaper that's only wet).

Most families use disposable diapers, which are inexpensive, hygienic, and easy. There's no advantage overall to more expensive brands. You'll find that different diapers fit differently, and you may need to experiment to find the best ones for your baby. Cloth diapers are another option, often using a diaper cover to keep them in place, though they are a bigger commitment than disposables.

No matter how frequently and carefully you change diapers, an occasional rash is going to happen. Treat rashes with extra naked time and an inexpensive diaper cream, one that contains about 20 percent zinc oxide. Talk to your pediatrician if your baby has frequent or difficult diaper rashes.

During every diaper change, keep a hand on your baby at all times. Newborns aren't typically rolling over or even trying to roll over, but if your baby is up on a changing table, you need to be careful. Steps for a successful change:

1. Get everything ready beforehand, ideally in a place that's comfortable for you to stand and get your job done. You need wipes, access to the diaper pail, diaper cream (maybe), a fresh diaper, and (often) spare clothes.

2. Remove clothes and then the soiled diaper. Try to keep feet out of the poo. This can be challenging; it helps to hold baby's feet up in the air with one hand while wiping with your other hand.

3. Clean the bottom, usually with a disposable wipe. You'll need to wipe enough to remove any poo. For an only-wet one, a quick swipe is plenty. Never scrub. For girl babies, you do not have to wipe way up in the vaginal area. For boys, you'll stay drier if you point his penis down or keep it covered. Place wipes in the soiled diaper, wrap the diaper tightly around itself with the tabs, and put it in the diaper pail.

4. Let your baby have some naked time. Fan with your hand. Sing a song.

5. Put on the new diaper, then clothes, then hand off baby or put them somewhere safe while you wash your hands. Repeat frequently.

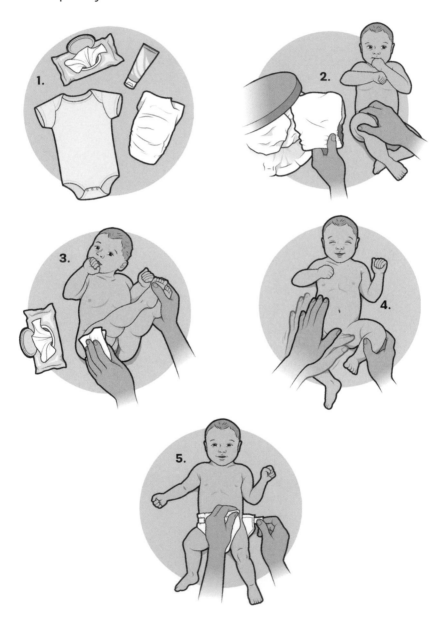

DIAPER BAG ESSENTIALS

You and your partner should keep a well-stocked diaper bag by the front door, ready for travel. Make sure to restock it as needed, and swap out clothes and diapers to the correct size as your baby grows. You'll need these items:

- Diapers, at least five, and maybe even include a few of the next size up.

- Diaper disposal bags, a few cheap, thin disposable bags (leftover takeout bags work great!) to wrap up soiled diapers in case you need a change without access to an appropriate trash. Please don't leave stinky diapers unwrapped in indoor trash receptacles, especially at your pediatrician's office. We have spare bags if you need them!

- At least one change of clothes.

- Diaper cream.

- Wipes, often in a smaller travel container.

- Hand sanitizer (better to wash with soap or water if available).

- A changing pad.

- Spare pacifier, bigger waterproof bags for clothes and things, spare blankets, burp cloths, bottles/nipples/feeding supplies if needed, nursing cover-up if needed.

- Also nice to have if you don't mind a bigger bag: spare shirts for you and your partner, bib for baby, a few first aid things, toys, hat, a little snack for parents, a cell phone backup battery, and some cash.

FEEDING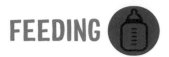

For your baby's best health, the AAP recommends exclusive breastfeeding for the first six months of life. However, bottle- and blended-fed babies can be super healthy, too. The most important thing is to ensure that your baby is well-fed either way. You should aim for a "responsive" feeding style—look for and respond to feeding and hunger cues—rather than aiming for a set schedule or set volumes of feeding. Newborn hunger cues include head turning (or "rooting") to find the breast, being alert and active, opening and closing the mouth, and sometimes crying.

BREASTFEEDING

Many women find breastfeeding (also called nursing) satisfying and fulfilling, but sometimes it's hard to get started. Work with your birth hospital's lactation service for support. They can help if things aren't going as smoothly as you'd like or just give you some good advice before you head home, especially for burping and soothing. Remember there are always options to keep both mom and baby safe and comfortable. Support your partner, whatever they decide, and especially if you have to change the plan.

Breastfeeding can lead to improved health for both baby and mother when it goes well. For instance, breastfed babies have fewer respiratory infections their first year, and mom will have a slightly lower lifetime risk of high blood pressure and some cancers. These risk differences are real but small. The best reason to breastfeed is that it's enjoyable and convenient for many families. However, if you and your partner decide to use infant formula sometimes or all the time, that can be the best decision for your family.

Breastfeeding should start ideally within a few minutes of your baby's birth. The early, first milk is called colostrum, and it's especially loaded with proteins and immunoglobulins to protect your baby's health. Your baby should try again frequently, at least every three hours for the first few weeks of life. Note that word, "try."

Some sessions won't go well, and that's okay. Mom should take a break and try again later. If your baby is awake one to two hours after the last feeding, mom should try again, especially if there are hunger cues.

A woman's milk supply depends on many things, and it takes time for milk to come in. The best way to increase supply is to empty both breasts frequently. If your baby is off to a rough start for any reason, they may not be emptying mom well. Talk with a lactation specialist and your pediatrician about pumping to help ensure a good supply. Pumped milk can be stored in a refrigerator or freezer for later use and can be a great way for dads to help with the caretaking. Even giving mom a break for one or two feedings can make a big difference.

Your role in breastfeeding will be to provide support for your partner. Breastfeeding requires a lot of time, hydration, calories, and energy. It can also wreak havoc on a mom's mental health if it's not going well, so be sure to check in with your partner and acknowledge what she may be experiencing. Keep plenty of healthy snacks on hand for her to eat while nursing, and make sure she's drinking plenty of water. Be as kind and encouraging as you can, and make her comfort a priority.

FORMULA FEEDING

Modern infant formula is specifically designed to provide good nutrition for newborns through age twelve months. It's very tightly regulated to ensure purity, consistency, and safety. There are a variety of formats. Ready-to-feed is premixed and easy, but over the long run it's much more expensive to use. There's also concentrated liquid available that must be mixed in the correct proportions with additional water. The most common and economical way to buy formula is powdered. Follow the exact instructions on the package to mix it correctly with water. There's a wide range of prices for infant formula. For the vast majority of babies, ordinary cow's milk formula works fine. More expensive formulas are not better in any important way.

There are some advantages to formula feeding. Both partners and the extended family can help feed directly. You'll know exactly how much is being taken, and you don't have to wait for mother's milk to come in. You don't have to breastfeed or bottle-feed exclusively; some families find it best to use a blend of both.

If you've decided to bottle-feed, begin immediately after birth, offering just an ounce or two. For the first two days of life, formula intake volumes may seem low as your baby adjusts and gets used to the outside world. A little spit-up is expected, but let your hospital team know it's going on.

As with breastfeeding, the best feeding style, especially at first, is responsive feeding both in timing and volume. Look for and respond to hunger cues to start feeds, and also look for signs that your baby has had enough. If they're turning away and not swallowing any- more, it's time to stop. Don't try to push more feeding on a baby who seems done.

CLUSTER FEEDING

Okay, you're chugging along, and your baby has been feeding about every two hours. Then one afternoon, bam, they want to eat every thirty minutes. You've probably run into a patch of cluster feeding. It can occur at any age.

We don't know exactly why babies cluster feed, but we do know it's more common in breastfed babies and often starts in the late afternoon or evening. During a cluster, your baby will show hunger cues and want to eat very frequently. They'll get upset if you push back and don't feed. A cluster may last an hour or so, and sometimes clusters of clusters occur, with more frequent feedings occurring off and on for a few days in a row.

During cluster feedings, babies seem well (they're only upset when they want to eat again). Though it may be tiring, you and your partner should feed through the cluster, responding to your baby's needs and giving them what they want. If you're concerned that your baby hasn't been getting enough or that feeding isn't going well, con- tact your pediatrician.

GAS, HICCUPS, AND SPIT-UP

Burping, gas, hiccups, spit-up—these are all normal things that every baby (and parent!) experiences. Your baby may be upset about these symptoms, especially at first, because they're not used to these feelings. They're new and weird, and to a little baby, that might cause worry. The best thing a parent of a newborn can do about these normal things is hold your baby and reassure them. Keep a sense of humor. Say "You sound like Mommy when you do that!" Try not to think about these things as medical problems that need medicine or need a medical solution. Hint: Farts will come more easily when your baby is relaxed.

BURPING YOUR NEWBORN

It's traditional to burp newborns, and I encourage you to try. It seems to help make some babies more comfortable. But it's not an essential skill. Some babies are hard to burp, and some babies get annoyed if you keep trying. The goal of a burp is to help make your baby feel better. If it's not helping, stop trying.

Burping should always be a gentle procedure, with little taps more than firm whaps. Try for only a minute or two or until a big burp comes up. You might want to have a burp cloth handy. The three most common and most successful burping positions are over the shoulder, on the lap, and across the lap (the belly flop).

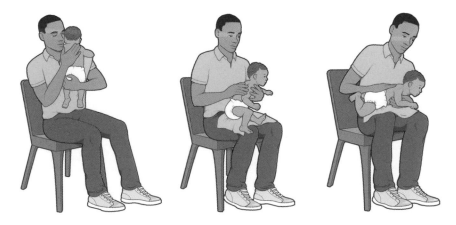

POOP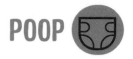

Your baby's first poops will be a different sort of stool called meconium. It's made of discarded cells and mucus, and it's very dark in color, almost black. It's quite sticky, too, and lacks odor. Sometimes babies will pass this first stool even before they're born.

Over the next few days, as your baby gets their first meals, meconium stools are passed frequently, usually at least four times a day. Then, by day three or four, the dark sticky stool will wash out and be replaced by a softer, yellow-to-greenish-colored poop. Breastfed babies tend to have more frequent, looser stools than formula-fed babies.

Stools that might cause concern would be very infrequent stools in the first two weeks of life, stools that remain black in color, stools that are bright red with blood, or stools that lack any color at all. If you're worried, talk with the nursery staff or your pediatrician.

Newborns will sometimes seem to strain with their poops. It's usually not because they're constipated or that the stool is too hard or thick to pass. More typically, it's because they haven't yet figured out how to relax their anus to pass stool. This is sometimes called "grunting baby syndrome" in the United Kingdom or "infant dyschezia" in the United States. It's not a lasting problem; babies get this figured out on their own. True constipation would be failure to pass any stool or stool that's hard or pebble-like. If your newborn is passing soft stool, even if they're making faces and grunting, it's not constipation.

SLEEPING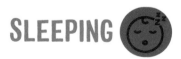

Newborns sleep a lot, usually around sixteen hours per twenty-four-hour cycle. It can be broken up between shorter naps and longer stretches, without a clear or consistent pattern, and can vary a lot from day to day. Usually, it's best to let sleeping babies sleep, though for the first two weeks, you'll probably be instructed to try to wake them if they haven't eaten in three hours. We'll talk more about specific sleep strategies for different ages in later chapters. For now, get the sleep you can, and try to help your partner get some sleep, too.

POSITIONING

There are very clear sleep positioning recommendations from the AAP, mirrored by just about every international children's health authority. To reduce the risk of sudden unexpected death, you should put your baby down to sleep flat on their back every time, not inclined. We don't know exactly why this is so crucial, but excellent studies have shown that this step alone reduces infant risk by at least half. You can reduce risks even further by following the steps for preventing sudden infant death syndrome on page 52.

Though you should place your baby down on their back, you should not use positioners, wedges, or anything else to force your baby to stay in that position. Those devices are not safe, because your baby could wriggle onto their side and suffocate. If you put your baby down flat on their back and they manage to squirm into another position, leave them there. You should also avoid crib bumpers, soft bedding, and anything else that could interfere with breathing.

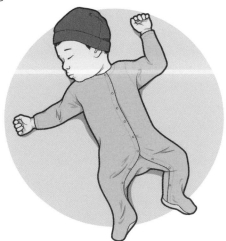

STARTLE REFLEX

One manifestation of a newborn's normal, immature brain is that they startle easily. The startle or Moro reflex can be triggered by a sound or motion. Your startled baby may throw back their head, extend their arms, and sometimes cry. This reflex reaction will gradually fade away, usually by two or three months. Some babies can be awakened by their own startle, disrupting sleep. You can try a nice safe swaddle to prevent the startle.

SWADDLING

Many babies find a swaddle—being wrapped up and limiting arm movement—to be relaxing and comforting. It can promote sleep, especially in premature babies or babies with an especially strong startle reflex. The AAP says swaddling is safe, as long as you do it correctly. You should stop swaddling when they start trying to roll over, typically at three to four months of life. Swaddling should keep the baby's arms fairly still but should never bind the legs. You can use a specially designed swaddle blanket or an ordinary receiving blanket like this:

1. Choose a soft blanket with a little stretch, and spread it out with one corner folded down.

2. Place baby's head above the fold.

3. Wrap first one side, with the arm extended (arm straight, pointing down).

4. Fold the extra blanket loosely up from the bottom.

5. Wrap the other arm, again while it's straight down, and use what's left of the tail of the blanket to wrap underneath the baby.

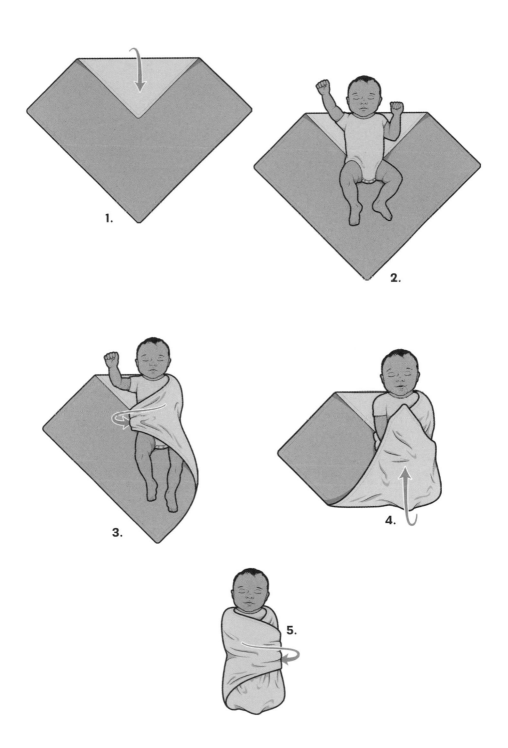

1.

2.

3.

4.

5.

PREVENTING SUDDEN INFANT DEATH SYNDROME

Sudden infant death syndrome (SIDS) refers to the sudden, unexpected, and unexplained death of a baby less than twelve months of age. We do not know the cause, but we do know steps that can reduce the risk dramatically. Improved knowledge and safer sleep have led to big drops in SIDS rates, from about 130 per 100,000 live births in 1990 to about 40 per 100,000 now. It's rare, and there are things you can do to make it even more rare, based on very solid evidence and recommendations from the AAP:

- Always put your baby down to sleep flat on their back, for naps and every sleep, every time, by everybody.

- Keep blankets, cushions, wedges, pillows, and anything soft out of the sleep environment.

- Have babies sleep on their own safe surface, not couches or recliners or their parents' bed.

- If babies fall asleep in a less safe place (like a car seat or the couch), move them to a safer environment as soon as practical.

- Do not use an inclined sleeper.

- Make sure your baby is fully vaccinated.

- Avoid exposure to secondhand smoke during pregnancy and after birth.

COLIC AND CRYING

All babies cry. I remember explaining to my oldest child when his younger brother was born that of course he was crying. He didn't know how to talk yet, and that was all he could say.

Sometimes babies cry because they're upset or distressed, or sometimes they cry to let off steam, or because (I think) they want to practice. If your baby is crying, think about a few other common possibilities: baby's hungry, too hot/cold, needs a burp or fart, needs a new diaper, or has a foot caught up and stuck in the onesie. If none of these possibilities seems to be the case, your baby may just be crying to let off some steam. With time, you and your partner will get very good at understanding your baby's different kinds of cries and what they mean.

Some babies cry a lot more than others. We sometimes call this colic. There's a formal definition of colic as an infant crying more than three hours a day, more than three days a week, for three or more weeks, but honestly, you're not going to find a pediatrician with a stopwatch. The definition we tend to use for colic is simpler: babies who cry too much, enough that it's worrying and exhausting the parents.

If your baby does a lot of crying, talk with their pediatrician. Review soothing methods, and try to arrange for some help from family or friends. The peak of colic is about six weeks, and it always gets better with time. Rarely, a medical condition can contribute to excessive crying. Your pediatrician is your best resource to sort this out. In the meantime, some earplugs or good noise-canceling headphones can help save your sanity.

A NOTE ON MILESTONES

A milestone, literally, is a stone marker beside the road, stating how far away the next thing is: "Ye Olde Pub, 2 miles." In pediatrics, we've come to use the term to label physical skills or behaviors that are expected to occur at a certain age. The current set of milestones, published in 2022, is keyed to the seventy-fifth percentile. In other words, seventy-five out of one hundred babies born at term will meet the milestone. Twenty-five out of one hundred will not, and that doesn't mean that those twenty-five babies have a medical problem.

The term "milestone" is misleading. The age of attaining skills varies for a lot of reasons, and it's not set in stone. Babies learn new skills at their own pace. Milestones can be helpful, but they're only one gauge of progress. They must be assessed as a whole, in context, rather than individually. Missing one milestone is not important; a pattern of overall delay can be a problem. Your pediatrician is the best person to keep an eye on your baby's developmental progress, through serial exams and checkups. If you're curious to view the complete set of milestones, look for "CDC Milestone Tracker" in an internet search, but don't let your baby's milestone progress get you down. Talk with your baby's pediatrician before you worry too much about milestones.

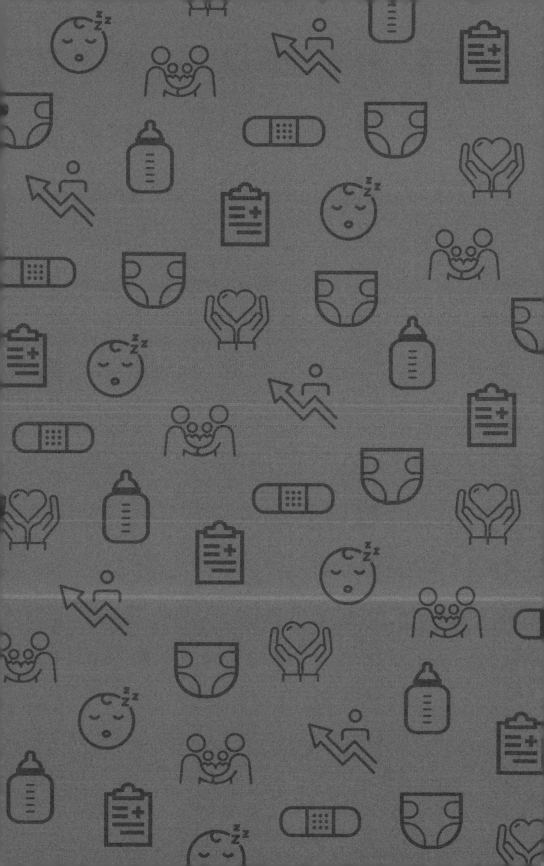

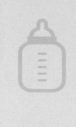

PART TWO

YOUR NEWBORN
IS HERE!

CHAPTER FIVE

THE FIRST WEEK WITH YOUR NEWBORN

Y ou've planned, you've prepped, you've waited, and now you're home. With your baby! Most full-term babies spend two to three days in the hospital, and that time goes quickly. It doesn't get more real than arriving home with all three of you for the first time.

In this chapter, we'll focus on your first week with baby. This is likely the biggest transition you've ever had to make in your life. We'll talk about your and your partner's physical and mental health and how to help support each other. You will be tired, and no one's getting much sleep yet, but together you're going to make it through this week. You'll become a more experienced and better dad with every passing day.

We'll also talk about your baby: what's changing and what they need to thrive. You've got baby's first medical visit this week, and we'll help you get prepared. It's a busy time!

LEAVING THE HOSPITAL

It's time to go home—you, your partner, and this little person you've just met. Your team will make sure mom and baby are healthy and safe and will give you extensive instructions on what to look for, who to call, and when to follow up.

To get home, you'll need clothes for your baby. (You and your partner need clothes too. You won't forget that.) You also need a car safety seat. Some birthing centers will insist you bring it up for inspection, making sure you know how to use it correctly. Mom will get to ride down to the car in a wheelchair, probably carrying baby in her arms. You'll drive up close for the pickup.

For that first car ride home, mom will probably ride in back with the baby, who'll be strapped facing backward in the secured safety seat. Some newborns might fuss at the unexpected position and new sights, though most are just fine. Many newborns even sleep through this ride. It's a new and exciting time for baby, too. You may want to bring a spare pacifier for the baby just in case there's fussing on the ride. And don't forget your favorite playlist or radio station!

You may or may not have someone at home to greet you, perhaps grandparents or the family dog. Do what works for you and mom. Don't feel that things have to be perfect or that you need to make sure that everything is done in a special, once-in-a-lifetime way. That's too much pressure on everyone. You and your baby have got years and years to get to know each other. Take some pictures (about ten thousand should do), and stay focused on keeping mom and baby comfortable.

YOUR PARTNER'S PHYSICAL AND MENTAL HEALTH AFTER BIRTH

Nothing is more important than the health of your family, which means both physical and mental health. No matter how well you've prepared, you're heading into a stressful time. Practice patience and flexibility, and keep a sense of humor. There will be some serious times and some worries, but there should also be time for smiling at the surprised look you'll get if you cluck like a chicken at your baby, too.

SUPPORT AFTER CHILDBIRTH

During pregnancy, mom had to put up with a lot of body changes. Some were positive, like that rosy glow. For many women, especially later in pregnancy, things are less positive. Pressure on the bladder pushing down and on the lungs pushing up. Trouble getting comfortable to walk, sleep, or eat. Acid reflux. Swollen toes. Your partner has already been dealing with some uncomfortable changes.

These don't all disappear quickly right after childbirth. It takes months for mom's uterus to recover and the swelling to go down. It also takes a long time for skin to return to its previous shape. Overall, it may be months or even years before her body feels like it did pre-pregnancy. Some changes are permanent, like stretch marks and C-section scars. You can best support your partner through these transitions by being there, physically and mentally. Communication is key. If you don't know how to help, ask. If she's overwhelmed and doesn't know what to tell you, ask her family and friends.

There may be some tangible ways you can help, like back or foot rubs. Keeping up on housework and preparing her meals and snacks can go a long way, too. But just as important is to understand and listen. Your partner knows it's going to take time to feel like herself again, and she's not expecting you to wave a magic wand. But she'll feel better knowing that you get it, so make sure she knows you appreciate all she's done to bring your baby into this world. She should know she's beautiful regardless of whether her body bounces back quickly or not.

PHYSICAL RECOVERY

Giving birth is almost certainly the most physically demanding thing your partner will ever do. For a vaginal birth, most moms remain very sore for at least a week or two. Sometimes there are lacerations or tears that will take longer to heal. Encourage your partner to work with her obstetric team to best address her recovery. She will almost certainly need to take some safe pain-relieving medication and will want to use ice packs and other methods to relieve soreness.

After a C-section, there's a different kind of soreness from the surgery. Pain medicine will be needed and will not harm a nursing baby. Most moms will be able to resume normal activities in four to eight weeks and shouldn't lift anything heavier than her baby for six to eight weeks or until cleared by her obstetrician.

Bathing can be tricky for moms after vaginal or C-section birth. Consider installing a showerhead with a handheld attachment to make it easier. Your job here is to keep communication open and help address practical things to help your partner's recovery. Bring ice. Keep pills organized, and give (gentle) reminders on the timing. Mom's going to be feeling some internal mental pressure to get up and do things that need to be done, even though she's sore. Help her out by doing those things yourself.

POSTPARTUM DEPRESSION AND ANXIETY

During the postpartum period—that's immediately after birth— many women experience symptoms like mood swings, crying spells, trouble sleeping, difficulty concentrating, and anxiety. In addition to putting up with physical pain and other symptoms, your partner is going through intense hormonal changes and dealing with the new emotional weight of keeping a newborn safe and fed. These symptoms often begin within a few days of childbirth and are most intense for the next two weeks. Having a temperamentally fussy baby or preexisting mental health challenges like an anxiety disorder may increase mom's risk of postpartum challenges, but postpartum depression can occur in anyone.

There's a lot on your shoulders, too. What you imagined was going to be a joyful period for you both may be punctuated with times of fear, sadness, exhaustion, or a lack of interest or motivation. Other negative emotions you both may feel can include irritability, anger, restlessness, or guilt and inadequacy. You're going through a huge change. Small things may make you emotional. You may be contemplating your future and your own life mission very differently and more profoundly now that you're a dad.

These feelings are common, and they're usually temporary and pass quickly. But if you or your partner are having these feelings intensely and especially if they're persistent, you should contact your physician or set up an appointment for a therapist. You're not alone in these feelings, and there is help.

Recurring thoughts of suicide or self-harm should be addressed immediately. Call the mental health crisis hotline at 988 for more info.

YOUR EMOTIONS AND MENTAL HEALTH

Men can experience a wide range of emotions with the birth of their baby. Many are very positive—a sense of pride, accomplishment, and maturity. You may feel a strong jolt of connection and love with your partner and your baby (but don't worry if this isn't an immediate feeling; it can take time). There can be some negative emotions, too. You might feel a little overwhelmed or inadequate or that you're having a hard time living up to what you expected to be able to do. Sleep deprivation is part of this. Remember that your body is suddenly processing a ton of stress without the rest and support it's used to. Mixed emotions are normal.

Don't put too much pressure on yourself. You're not going to be perfect, and some things that you didn't expect to be challenging might end up being big stumbling blocks. You might feel awkward at first, holding and caring for a tiny baby. That will get better, and it will feel more natural soon. You have the rest of your life to be a dad. You don't need to figure it out in a week.

You might also start to worry about balancing work and career and financial goals. There's time for that later. Stay in the present, with what you and your partner and your baby need now. You can't predict the future, so stop trying to anticipate it using what little energy you have.

You'll be busy with a lot to do. Self-care is important. You need to eat and sleep. An exhausted, strung-out dad isn't going to be able to help out as much with mom and baby. This doesn't mean you sleep and mom doesn't. Find a system that works for you both, whether it's splitting the night into shifts, taking turns napping during the day, or having a friend or family member occasionally help out overnight or in the mornings.

Take some time to share how you're feeling with your partner, your family, and your closest friends. Share the good news and the positive times but the challenges, too. Be honest. You'll see that other dads have also been through this. And if things are really overwhelming you to the point you or others feel concerned, check in with a professional.

WEEK ONE MILESTONES

For this first week, the theme will be adapting. Your baby is adapting to a dramatically changed world. So are you.

A few days ago, your baby had only known life upside down, underwater, and squeezed tight. There was no feeling of air on their skin and no sensations of swallowing and digestion and gas bubbles and passing stool. No lights, either. Any sounds were muffled and distant.

Then, suddenly, lights and sounds and eating and that weird feeling of clothes on skin. The first week is all about adapting, and there's a lot for the baby to get used to. Expect schedules and reactions to be inconsistent, with periods of crying and confusion (maybe for you and your partner, too).

Physically, babies will lose weight for the first few days of life. This is expected and normal. Weight should start inching back upward by day five, gaining about an ounce a day. Other measurements, like length and head circumference, are less accurate and don't track neatly in the short run.

Your baby will move and wiggle when awake and even a bit while asleep. Arms and legs should all move. If you notice a persistent lack of movement or different-looking movement in one extremity, bring it to the doctor's attention. Most of the time, newborns like to stay kind of curled up, with bent elbows and bent knees. You might also notice some tremors or rapid shaking of arms or feet or the chin. With your gentle touch, this will stop. It's not a problem. Your baby is practicing moving and feeling what movement is like.

Newborns can see and hear, too. The best focus will be about a foot away from their eyes. They can't yet track your movement, but while awake, their eyes will move together and rarely cross. Newborns can hear, too, but they can't tell where sound is coming from yet, so don't expect your baby to turn their head toward sounds.

BONDING

Bonding isn't just another job you have to do. Instead, think about it as a reward—your relaxation time. There's no one way you have to do this, no exact frequency or number of hours. You may prefer something quiet (like skin-to-skin time), running errands together, or just sitting and talking. The most important thing is that you find this time with your baby relaxing. Do what *you* like.

Time for bonding can include holding and walking around, explaining, and talking about the house. Or it could include singing or (gently) dancing. It could be sitting outside in a rocker, enjoying the sounds of nature together, or maybe going together to the hardware store to find the right valve to fix a leaking faucet. Any or all these things and more are great times to build lasting bonds.

Skin-to-skin time is great, too, though perhaps not in the plumbing aisle. Traditionally this is done with a naked baby lying on a parent's bare chest, maybe under a blanket. Diapers are optional but probably a good idea (are you feeling lucky?).

Frequent bonding times are encouraged, whether in long stretches or little snippets, whether scheduled or when you find a quiet moment. It's all good.

IT'S OKAY IF YOU'RE NOT FEELING A BOND

Bonding with your newborn may begin early and progress quickly, or it may start a little later and move more slowly. You may not sense a strong attachment with your baby until weeks or months after birth. How quickly bonds develop depends on you and your partner's health and outlook, outside pressures and distractions, your baby's personality, and your own life experiences and expectations.

Many new parents feel a lot of pressure to develop a bond immediately, but that's not always realistic or even possible. Try not to feel anxious or guilty if you don't connect right away. Share how you feel with your partner and perhaps your parents or your child's doctor. You'll see that you're not alone. Bonding is not a onetime process or something that must take place at a certain time or in a certain way. Like a tall and sturdy tree, lasting bonds can take time to grow.

No matter how you feel about your baby, you must help with their care. They don't know what to think about you, either. Magical moments will come in time, but for now, try to provide the best care you can regardless of how you feel.

SOOTHING

Those big adaptations needed after birth are going to lead to some fussy periods, times when your baby is a little anxious and not sure about what's going on. No matter their personality—and they do already have their own personality—there will be times when any newborn is going to need to blow off some steam.

The best response is calm reassurance. If your baby continues to fuss after checking the diaper and seeing if it's time for a meal, here are some good soothing ideas to try. Some will work better than others. You'll learn what your baby likes best.

- **Swaddling:** See page 50.

- **Swaying:** The key here is a gentle walk and sway in a natural sort of rhythm. Singing or talking is an optional add-on to these times.

- **Shushing:** Again, gentle and reassuring. You're not arguing or telling them to be quiet. You're saying, "It's okay. I know things seem scary now. I got you."

- **Sights and sounds:** As in a change of scene. Need something at the grocery store? Or maybe just visit the basement and explain how a drill press works.

Tip: You and your partner have to take turns here. You can't always be the soother. Sometimes, in fact, you will need to be the "soothee." If both adults need a break, it's okay to put a fussy baby down and take a breather. No harm done.

FEEDING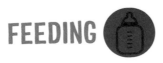

Based on your baby's birth weight, health, and other factors, you may get more specific feeding instructions from the birth hospital or your pediatrician. Follow those. Here are some general guidelines.

Newborns should be offered their next meal two to three hours after the beginning of the previous meal. Even earlier if your baby is awake and showing hunger cues like rooting around, acting especially active, or making mouth-smacking movements. If your baby is sleeping soundly at the two-hour mark, let them sleep, but if awake, now's the time to start the next feeding. At three hours, if still asleep, try to wake baby up.

Overall, breastfed babies should feed a little more frequently, especially as mom's milk is coming in at first. But frequent breast-feeding doesn't have to mean long breastfeeding. It usually takes fifteen to twenty minutes on each side, then it's time for a break. Hour-long nursing sessions are exhausting for everyone. It's better to get both breasts emptied than to spend too much time on the first side. Save some energy (and time) for the other side, even if that means breaking the seal to pop the baby off and swapping over before they seem done.

Babies who are exclusively or mostly breastfed should also be given a vitamin D supplement containing 400 International Units (IU) once a day. Use an over-the-counter supplement, following the dosing instructions on the label.

For formula-fed babies, again aim for two to three hours from the beginning of one feeding to the next. If your baby is asleep and it's time for a meal, prepare the bottle first, or work as a team (dad preps, mom wakes, or vice versa). Newborn feeding volumes often start as low as one ounce (thirty milliliters) at first and get up to the one to two ounce range by the end of the first week (thirty to sixty milliliters). A little more is okay, too, but might lead to more spitting up. You'll want to prepare a bottle with a little more volume than you expect your baby to take. If they don't finish it, that's okay. Dump the leftovers, and start fresh next time.

WEEK ONE: HEALTHY POOP

Newborn poop undergoes a lot of changes that first week. It starts as blackish-green, sticky meconium. The first poops can be difficult to wipe off. Within about four days, the meconium will wash out, and you'll see a transition to a much softer, runnier stool. The color can be anywhere on the rainbow from bright yellow to green to brown.

You will probably see a lot of poop this first week, four or more a day. Some will be more like little streaks, and some will be bigger. They'll be soft, not formed, and won't have much of an odor yet.

SLEEPING

There's a wide range of "normal" sleep amounts for a newborn. Most will sleep a total of fourteen to seventeen hours a day and sometimes more. Some of the sleep will be in longer stretches, two or maybe even three hours at a time. Some of it will be in short catnaps. Most pediatricians don't ask parents to track or record sleep patterns—you've got enough other things to do—but if you're worried, you can keep a log for a few days to share with your pediatrician.

A typical pattern for newborns is the sleep-eat-play cycle. When they wake from a nap, it's time for a meal. Afterward, there can be a little bit of quiet and alert bonding or playtime before the next nap. But this pattern is often hard to rely on, especially early on. Your baby may not want to eat immediately after waking. Or they might wake, eat, stay up a bit, eat again, and fall asleep during the meal. Or take one breast, nap a bit, then wake up and want the other one. Especially this first week, roll with the changes, and don't expect consistency. You're all getting used to each other. The most important thing now isn't trying to track or force sleep. Just provide a safe sleep environment (see page 49), and don't pressure yourself or your baby to follow a schedule or pattern.

HELPING YOUR NEWBORN SLEEP

Sleep is hard. You may have thought that people have an instinctive ability to fall asleep and stay asleep and to go to sleep when they're tired. Nope. These are skills that your baby needs to learn, and it will take time.

Though you cannot make a baby sleep, there are things you can do to help reinforce and build good sleep skills:

- **Show them the difference between day and night.** Keep lights on during the day and dim or off at night. Play and talk more during the day. At night, it's all business, without added stimulation from a lot of talking and activity.

- **Direct eye contact is stimulating for babies.** Avoid prolonged eye contact during nighttime feedings and changes. Yes, it's cute that they stare at you, but don't stare back. It's all business at night.

- **Look for sleep cues,** and put baby down *before* they're super tired. Exhausted babies will have a harder time making the transition to sleep.

- **Get your baby used to being put down.** This is a difficult step. Babies fall asleep quickly, and you'll be reluctant to put them down because that may wake them up again. It's okay. Try. If you never try to put them down, it will take much longer to get good long stretches of sleep.

- **Work toward a consistent routine.** Start working on the sleep setting early. This can involve a going-to-sleep song, a soothing white noise generator, and a specific room or place for sleep that the baby can grow to depend on.

THE FIRST PEDIATRICIAN VISIT

The AAP recommends a first in-person visit with your baby's pediatrician two to three days after you go home. Sometimes, your pediatrician may have already visited you in the hospital. Or perhaps your hospital or birthing center used an in-house provider for the initial stay.

If there were any concerns in the hospital, you may have been instructed to see the pediatrician earlier, even one day after discharge. Please follow those instructions, and try to call the pediatrician's office to set up an early appointment ASAP. Early appointments are often driven by a need to recheck jaundice, feeding, or weight concerns.

At the first visit, I try to see how parents and any siblings are doing first. There's a lot going on, and we don't want simple things to fall through the cracks.

Expect a lot of questions about feeding and poop, a careful assessment of growth and vital signs, and a complete and naked physical exam (the baby, I mean). Lots of changes and adaptations are occurring, and we need to check especially the circulatory system, bones and joints, and skin.

Most important, parents need to get their questions answered. You may want to bring a printed or handwritten list of the questions that are essential to you. They're all good questions, but they're no good if you don't ask them! We're used to new parents, and we love to talk about new babies, so fire away. This is your time with the best expert available to make sure all is well and keep your family on the healthiest path.

CHAPTER SIX

THE FIRST MONTH WITH YOUR NEWBORN

You're a dad now, and your home and your family are changing. Your baby has started to settle in, getting used to life outside the womb. By the end of the first month, your baby is more alert and responsive. And they're just starting to learn!

In this chapter, we'll tackle the first month, including physical and developmental changes to expect and how to best help take care of your baby, your partner, and yourself. We'll talk about feeding, pooping, and sleeping. Those three topics will remain a big focus of your life as the parent of a young baby.

There are more changes coming, more challenges and new things for you and your baby to learn. You've gotten off to a good start, and being a dad is starting to feel more natural. Maybe you're even starting to feel like it's more than a job. It's you.

GROWTH AND APPEARANCE

Babies by the end of their first month have usually gained about one to two pounds over birth weight, plus an inch or so of length. That may not sound like much, but it means many have outgrown that first set of clothes and the newborn baby diaper size. You can tell by holding your baby that they're a little more solid, with better head control and stronger muscles. Their cheeks will fill in, and their little legs will feel stronger and more substantial.

By about two weeks of life, the umbilical cord will fall off. After that happens, you can start regular tub baths, filling up the sink insert about halfway so your baby is about half-dunked in the water. Your baby's skin may be sensitive. If there are dry patches, you'll want to use a nice, thick, oily moisturizer after baths.

Many babies lose a lot of their hair by the end of the first month. It will all grow back in, though maybe with a little different color or texture. You'll see!

Newborn eye color is often darkish blue or a slate-gray color, or it may be varying shades of brown at first. The color will change over the first year or so, and subtle changes can even occur later. After twenty-five years of greeting newborns, I still can't guess what their later eye color will be. It's yet another "You'll see!"

Both boy and girl babies can have some breast swelling, sometimes only on one side. This is normal. Of course, if you're concerned about anything related to your baby's body or appearance, talk with their pediatrician. That's your best resource.

MOVEMENT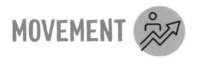

By the end of the first month, your baby's movement will be smoother and more coordinated. They're still learning, though. Their arms and legs will move with a somewhat jerky quality, sometimes with quivering or a tremor. Hands will be brought toward the face, especially toward the eyes and mouth, often held in tight fists. Your baby will start to support their head, bringing it up against gravity, but only for a moment before flopping back down. You'll still want to give some head support.

You'll also want to give your baby a chance to get a little exercise with tummy time. While awake, for a few minutes at a time, let them rest on their chest and tummy. They'll move their head from side to side, though they won't yet be able to arch up or support their chest on extended arms. That comes later. If your baby's getting upset, pick them back up. That's how they tell you they've had enough tummy time for now.

Your one-month-old will still show normal newborn reflexes in their movement. These include grasping tightly if something touches their palm (the grasping reflex), turning their head to a stroke of the cheek (rooting), and startling to sound or sudden movements (the Moro reflex). There are other newborn reflexes that your pediatrician can demonstrate for you. Most of these start to gradually fade away by four to six months as the nervous system matures.

RETURNING TO WORK

United States federal law—the Family and Medical Leave Act, or FMLA—requires most larger employers to give new dads at least twelve weeks of unpaid leave. Some employers may be more generous, but that's all you're guaranteed. Even then, this may not apply to you, and that loss of income may be a big problem for many families.

Still, as best you can, try to make the most of this first twelve weeks. It's an important time for moms to recover physically and for families to bond and get into the rhythm of working as a team. It won't feel like enough time (and probably isn't), but it's important not to give in to guilt or shame. Your goal should be getting to know your baby as much as you can so that you can develop bonds that last.

There will be competing expectations and demands on your time, and you should be realistic about what you can and cannot do. Good communication and honesty with both your work team and your family will help. It's a delicate balancing act that no one does perfectly. Extend honesty to yourself, and determine what your priorities are, then set goals around those. Don't do what you think others would do or would want you to do. It can help to have an advance plan, perhaps starting with part days or flexible time to ease back into work. Try to focus on your core responsibilities first rather than on everything you could possibly do or everything you used to do.

SENSORY DEVELOPMENT

Your baby is becoming more interested in exploring the world with their senses. By now, some visual preferences have emerged. Many babies like to look at black-and-white or high-contrast images and human faces. Their focus remains best at about a twelve-inch distance, and their eyes should always move together, though not consistently adjusting to track a moving target quite yet.

Your baby's sense of hearing is quite good. Even quiet noises can be heard and will sometimes trigger a reaction. Your baby will start turning their head when there's noise, though not consistently toward a sound.

Smell and touch sensation is a little more difficult to assess day by day, but from research settings, we know one-month-olds prefer sweet tastes and the scent and taste of their own mother's breast milk. Babies seem happier with soft touch sensations and gentle handling.

FEEDING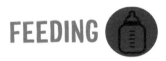

You've settled into a feeding style by now, perhaps at the breast, perhaps using a bottle of pumped milk or formula, or perhaps a blend. None of these are always the "best" way. You should do what works for everyone, including mom and baby. Don't feel bad if your feeding style is different from what you imagined it would be, and don't pressure mom into a change that isn't what she wants or isn't healthy for her or baby.

By one month of age, babies using a bottle are taking about three to four ounces per feeding, typically six to eight times a day. Most babies are getting up a few times for night feeds, though you do not have to wake them as they start sleeping longer. No other nutrition is needed now, other than mother's milk and/or commercial baby formula. Don't add cereal to bottles, and always make sure you're mixing formula by following the exact directions on the package.

All babies spit up. The spit-up will look more or less like swallowed milk, or it may have separated into curds and whey, with clear liquid mixed with some white strands or clumps. Normal spitting up is painless, and your baby should stay happy and feeding well. If you think there's excessive or painful spit-up, talk with your baby's doctor.

All babies have gas, too. They fart and burp and make all kinds of noises. Burping helps some but isn't essential and is never 100 percent effective. Your best response to a gassy baby is to keep a sense of humor. Hold and reassure your baby that these feelings are normal and part of life. Bottle-fed babies experiencing lots of gas may benefit from a change in bottle style or nipple shape. It can also help to use the soothing techniques from page 67.

Questions often come up about whether the milk itself is causing problems. For formula-fed babies, almost all ordinary formula is cow's milk–based, and they're all essentially identical. It won't hurt to swap or try different brands if you'd like. If your baby is having health problems, your pediatrician may recommend a specific formula, often one called "hypoallergenic" that is made with broken-down proteins.

Some people also recommend dietary restrictions for nursing moms to reduce gas or fussiness for the baby. This is rarely a good idea. Restrictions don't usually help and can lead to more misery and guilt. Moms work hard and should eat the foods they like. Dads, too! If your baby is especially fussy or gassy, get advice from your pediatrician.

MONTH ONE: HEALTHY POOP

Newborns poop frequently, but as they reach one month they poop less and less. Some breastfed babies may go many days between poops. As long as it's soft and painless when it does come out, that's not constipation, and it's not a problem.

You'll also see changes in color, consistency, and odor as your baby matures and normal bacteria begin colonizing the gut. The color and consistency can change from day to day. Overall, a normal one-month poop should remain on the rainbow of color from yellow to green to brown and be about as soft as applesauce.

SLEEPING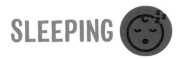

You're tired. Your partner is tired. Your baby is tired. So why aren't you sleeping better? It's because good sleep for babies is a learned skill. It is not automatic. Babies don't automatically sleep just because they're tired.

An absolute rule of parenting is that you can't make your baby sleep. What you can do is set the stage to improve your chances of successfully transitioning to independent, long stretches of sleep. There are still no guarantees. Some babies are born with good sleep skills and are easy to train; others will fight you at every step. You can do everything "right" and still struggle. If anyone says "just do this thing, it always works," they're not being realistic.

Your goal for this first month should be improved sleep. You'll want to get to some longer stretches and at least an outline of a schedule that works for the family. Don't be too rigid or set the bar too high.

For the first month, most babies will sleep a total of fourteen to seventeen hours over each twenty-four-hour period. Wake times usually last thirty to ninety minutes and tend to get longer as the day goes on (that is, morning wake periods are often shorter, with longer stretches in the later afternoon). Naps can be erratic, with some short and some long, from thirty minutes to two hours. You'll see patterns emerging by about two weeks, with similar-length naps at similar times, but they're not set in stone or even set in wet concrete. More like set in Jell-O, if that makes sense. There's wiggling and shifting and surprises, and just when you think you've got it nailed down, another change.

Should you wake a sleeping baby? Yes, at first. Until your baby gets back to birth weight, it's a good idea to wake them if it's been three hours since the start of their last feed.

By the two-week checkup, most babies are past their birth weight. My advice, unless there are medical issues, is to stop night waking at around two weeks. Let your baby sleep as long as they want to (once you get your pediatrician's okay that all is well).

My advice for day napping is the same: Usually past the two-week checkup, don't wake a sleeping baby during the day, either. That might sound counterintuitive. You might think, "If I get my baby up more during the day, we'll get longer naps and longer night stretches." In my experience, this doesn't work. Babies who are woken up get strung out and upset and don't sleep well. Rested babies sleep better. Remember, it's not tiredness that drives babies to sleep; it's a learned skill. You can help them learn better by letting them sleep, even if it's not convenient for your desired schedule.

One way to help nudge babies toward better sleep is to feed them as soon as they wake up. Follow a repeating pattern of sleep, eat, then play (then sleep again). The key here is to try not to use the "eat" step as a cue to fall asleep again. Instead, have some playtime after a meal, and then put your baby down to sleep, ideally before they're super tired or upset or exhausted. Again, they need to learn to sleep, and learning is easier when they're not fussy or upset. Separating "eat" from "sleep" will make later, more active sleep training easier, quicker, and more successful. This cycle won't work every time. Think of it as a goal, and try not to get frustrated when your baby strays from your plan.

MENTAL AND SOCIAL DEVELOPMENT

Your baby's brain grows dramatically during their first months of life. That means big steps in all the stuff that brains do, including thinking and planning. Thought pathways, or brain synapses, are being created and modified at a dizzying rate.

What you'll see over the first month includes the development of communication skills. Your baby will not be talking yet, but communication is starting. By one month, babies will kind of gurgle and seem happy when they're content. They'll enjoy looking at parents' faces and will share your moods. If you're cranky, they'll get cranky, and if you're happy, that will often rub off on them, too. They'll calm when you pick them up, especially if you hold and rock and talk with a slow, gentle rhythm. Sharing moods and experiences is a first step to communication and helps build family bonds.

Babies cry a lot, especially at first. Try not to think of crying as always expressing sadness or a negative mood. To a baby, sometimes crying is more of a reflex or a way to work through stress. It's a form of inexact communication. Over time, they'll learn to use crying more precisely to say something specific. For now, like the little smile with gas or a surprised pout, crying is a communication skill to practice.

Different phases or moods of awake time call for different interactions. When your baby is quiet and alert, maybe right after a feeding, it's a great time to talk and hold and let your baby see how your facial expressions convey what's going on. If your baby is getting a little cranky, you might walk around and try to distract a little. During crying time, your main approach should be to hold and reassure so your baby knows they're safe and it's okay to cry. Don't argue with them. Saying "Don't cry" is unlikely to help. Instead, agree with their mood, and tell them "It's okay, buddy. I got you. I'm listening."

HOW TO PLAY

Your play style should depend on what both you and your baby like. A good rule of thumb: If you and your baby are enjoying it, keep doing it! Here are some ideas to get started.

- **Talk.** Tell stories, and use facial expressions and sound effects and anything else that comes to mind.

- **Make funny or weird faces, and explain what you're doing.** "This is what I look like when I eat a spicy taco!"

- **Take your baby on a "world tour."** Keeping in mind that your baby is small and their world is small, a world tour is a stroll around your home, explaining rooms and appliances and where you've hidden the doughnuts. The world tour of course can include your neighborhood or the local coffee shop. Talk about the things you see and the people you meet.

MONTH ONE WELL VISIT

During your baby's first month, you'll be seeing a lot of their pediatrician. That's because changes occur rapidly, and this is a time when we need to keep an eye on things. There are also a lot of questions to answer and concerns to discuss, so take advantage of these appointments, come prepared, and be ready to ask everything that's on your mind. Feel free to bring a paper list or read off notes and questions from your phone. Do whatever you need to make sure you've got your questions answered.

Typical first visits for a healthy baby are at a few days after being discharged from the hospital, two weeks, and one month of life. At each visit, your baby will be weighed and measured and will receive a thorough examination. Pediatricians look, listen, feel, and run through a mental checklist of hundreds of things we've seen before. We'll talk about growth, feeding, sleep, and poop, and make sure everything is on track.

Here are a few of the more common questions:

- Is the baby eating and growing enough?

- Are they developmentally on track?

- How can we get them to sleep more?

MILESTONES AND MEDICAL CONCERNS

Apart from questions about growth, sleep, eating, and poop, a few other common medical concerns come up at the two-week and one-month visits. None of these are serious, and all usually resolve on their own.

- **Scalp scale:** Usually "cradle cap" clears up on its own, or you can help it along with a gentle oil massage and a soft baby brush.

- **Peeling skin:** Not a concern. This happens from the transition to the outside, dry world.

- **Dry skin:** Best treated with moisturizing ointment.

- **Watery or gunky eyes:** Caused by blocked tear ducts. Let us know right away if the white of the eye is red; otherwise, this isn't a big concern. Just wipe them with a warm, soft towel.

However, if you see any of these things frequently, mention them to your pediatrician:

- Slow feeding with a poor or inconsistent suck

- Doesn't react to bright lights by closing eyes

- Doesn't startle or react to loud noises

- Doesn't focus and follow a close object that's moving in their line of sight

- Seems especially stiff or not moving limbs freely and equally

- Seems excessively loose or floppy, like a rag doll

PARTNER CHECK-IN

Take a step back. Think a moment about all that's changed and all that's still changing. It's been quite a roller coaster, and no matter how supportive you've been and how smoothly (or less smoothly) things have gone, your partner has been through a lot. Her body changed in all kinds of ways and isn't back to the way it was, she's got all kinds of raging hormones screaming at her from the inside, and she's exhausted.

Your partner knows you can't solve everything, and she doesn't expect you to. The most important thing is to be there. Physically, mentally, and emotionally, be ready to share and listen. Offer back or foot rubs. Do her share of the chores. Let her sleep.

Maybe even more important: Run interference with nosy neighbors or troublesome relatives who aren't helping build your partner up. Be supportive. Talk about the funny moments, the good times, and what you're looking forward to. Offer encouragement, and tell her what a great job she's doing.

Be mindful of postpartum depression, too. The "baby blues" are a common side effect of all the physiological changes she's endured, but lasting, persistent depression and despair are not. If she seems resentful, detached, or unwilling to care for the baby, it's time to have a conversation about professional help.

SELF CHECK-IN

You're going to need to check in on yourself, too. You are working hard, with at least one extra job that's new and exciting and scary. You're supporting your partner and helping with the baby. I'll bet you sometimes feel stretched pretty thin.

Think about your time, what really energizes you, what relaxes you, and what you might miss now that your life has changed. There is at least a little time for your own pleasures and distractions. However, you cannot force your old life into your new one. The goal here is to identify what you most enjoy and then modify it to fit your new reality. Love football? You can probably make that fantasy league work, but don't expect to watch every game, every Sunday. There may be hobbies and relationships and dive bars you need to say goodbye to.

And while it may be fun to burn the midnight oil on a gaming session or streaming marathon, you'll never, ever regret getting extra sleep.

CHAPTER SEVEN

THE SECOND MONTH WITH YOUR NEWBORN

I t's your family's second month together, and the theme is now routines. You've got a loose schedule or routine in place, with meals and naps happening around the same time every day. Of course, your baby can't tell time yet, so be ready for surprises!

In this chapter, we'll cover this second month: how your baby looks and acts, how they move and perceive the world, and what kinds of games and activities will be fun for you both. We'll update feeding and sleeping routines and tell you how to keep your baby, your partner, and yourself feeling strong and confident. You're an experienced dad now, with more to learn. Hopefully the first month gave you a sense you can do this. If not, just hang in there. You and your baby are growing, together!

GROWTH AND APPEARANCE

During this second month, your baby will grow another one to one and a half inches and gain about two pounds. These are only estimates. Your pediatrician will be tracking your baby's growth and will let you know if there are concerns. It never hurts to ask.

One thing to keep in mind with measurements of length: Babies are squirmy, and they don't like to be held down to check their size. Often, length measurements are a little off and aren't super accurate if repeated. All we want to see early on is a general upward trend.

Weights, on the other hand, can be measured quite accurately. A graph of your baby's overall weight gain will track neatly on the chart, following the percentile curves. Again, ask your pediatrician to go over your baby's growth numbers if you're especially interested or concerned.

Some days, you'll pick up your baby in the morning and think, "Did you grow?" It isn't your imagination. Both height and weight increase unevenly, in spurts, some days far more than others. Over the course of several weeks, it all evens out.

Babies are born with disproportionately big heads (compared with older children or adults). Those heads keep growing rapidly, by about half an inch in circumference each month. Though some heads may be a little misshapen at birth, by now your baby's head should be round and should continue to grow round and symmetric.

MOVEMENT

During your baby's second month, movements will continue to become smoother and more coordinated. Arms and legs on both sides should move equally well.

By the end of the second month (that is, by the two-month birthday), a baby placed on their tummy will be starting to push up with their arms to get the chest and back up off the floor or table. The head can usually be raised to about forty-five degrees and will turn from side to side as your baby looks around. They won't hold that position for very long. It's good exercise to practice this tummy time.

During the second month, your baby will start loosening their hands, too, rather than clenching them into little fists most of the time. They'll wrap their fingers around an object to grab it and won't want to let go. They'll also clasp their hands together and sometimes bring their hands to their mouth. That may be a clue that they're getting hungry.

Some babies will soothe themselves by sucking on one or more fingers or their hand or a knuckle. I would not discourage this. Being able to settle yourself is a great life skill for babies to achieve. If your baby is making progress toward self-soothing by sucking their fingers, it's fine.

SENSORY DEVELOPMENT

Your baby's eyesight is getting sharp, and they're better able to focus on objects and faces. Colors are becoming more vibrant, and they're more interested in looking at contrasting or bright shapes. Their eyes should track, moving smoothly to follow you as you move slowly from side to side or up and down. Most of the time, when your baby is awake with their eyes open, they'll be looking directly at something rather than letting their eyes wander.

Hearing has gotten better, too. Your baby may react differently to the sounds of different people's voices and will sometimes try to turn their head to zero in on who's speaking. Loud and unexpected noises can still startle them, but their exaggerated whole body startle is starting to fade.

FEEDING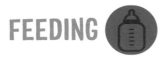

Nursing babies are still feeding frequently, eight or more times in a twenty-four-hour period. With some luck and gentle nudging, you can get some longer stretches at night. The best strategy here is to try to keep daytime feedings close together. If it's been more than two hours since the start of the last daytime feeding and your baby is awake, start the next feeding. At night, let your baby sleep as long as they can. When they wake up, feed them.

Babies who are exclusively nursing or mostly nursing should take a vitamin D supplement, 400 IU once a day.

Formula-fed babies tend to space out feedings a little more than breastfed babies at this age. They'll usually take something like five to six ounces at a time in about six bottles a day (babies who take smaller bottles have more frequent feeds).

Avoid bottle propping. Don't use a blanket or toy or anything else to hold a bottle vertically for hands-free feeding. Babies should be in a semi-upright position while bottle-feeding to reduce the risk of ear infections and other health hazards.

For both bottle-fed and nursing babies, watch for hunger cues. They're more important to guide your day than the exact scheduled time. Feeding schedules at this age are a good idea, but think of them as a general goal. They're not firm or set in stone. Some days, your baby will want to feed more or less frequently or at odd times. Roll with it.

Your baby doesn't need any other nutrition at this age. Just breast milk and extra vitamin D, infant formula, or a blend of these. Don't give any extra water, and don't add cereal or anything else to the bottle. This won't help your baby sleep better and won't help with gas or spitting up.

Both gas and reflux discomfort should start to improve by now. Your baby has started to figure out, with your reassurance, that these unexpected and weird feelings are not so unexpected or weird anymore. There will still be spit-up and farts and burps but now with less drama and even a few smiles.

COLIC AND CRYING

Though crying with gas and spit-up is improving, normal babies still do a lot of crying at this age. It's often concentrated in the evening during a consistent time, say from 7:00 to 9:30 p.m. During this time, your baby will cry a lot. They'll be briefly consolable by holding or rocking or feeding but will start crying again every few minutes. Technically, if there's more than three hours of crying more than three days in a week, it's called colic, but any baby who cries more than expected, without an apparent medical cause, is called colicky.

Colicky crying peaks at six weeks of life and then improves. Your pediatrician is your best resource to evaluate your baby to see if there's any medical cause or medical intervention needed. A crying baby can be extra exhausting for you and your partner. Take turns holding and soothing. Look to friends and family to come over and help some evenings so you can get a break. Wireless earbuds playing podcasts or playlists or even just earplugs can help you maintain your sanity while you soothe your baby during these seemingly endless cry-a-thons.

MONTH TWO: HEALTHY POOP

As your baby passes their first-month birthday, a dramatic change can happen with poop frequency. Stools can go from several times a day to just once a day, once every other day, or even once every five days. The change is most dramatic with breastfed babies. I've seen them go from ten poops a day to once every ten days, and it's all normal!

A truly constipated baby will pass little hard rocks or pellets of poop or poop squeezed into a ribbon-like shape. Even if your baby's poop isn't frequent, it's normal as long as it's soft when it does arrive.

SLEEPING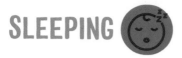

Sleep is almost certainly at the top of your "I wish I could fix this" list. It has gotten better but not by much. Your baby is still sleeping fourteen to seventeen hours a day and should have somewhat longer stretches at night. But very few babies this age are sleeping all the way through the night on their own. Most are still up two times or more and often need to eat to get back to sleep again.

Now is not the time to get strict about sleep training. Some babies will sleep better and longer than others, no matter what you do. Still, there are gentle things you can do to encourage longer stretches at night:

- **Be consistent about your bedtime routine.** This can include bathing, massage, and maybe reading together. Whatever you do, do the same things in the same order at the same time every night.

- **Be consistent about where your baby falls asleep.** In their own crib or bassinet, placed on their back, is safest and best.

- **Use other sleep cues.** These may include a white noise machine or a pacifier, again in the same place at the same time.

- **Try to put your baby down *before* they fall asleep.** This is tricky—babies quickly fall asleep in your arms, and you'll miss the transition sometimes. That's okay. Just put your sleeping baby down on their back if that happens. But try, at least some-times, to get your baby down while still awake.

- **Do not wake your baby at night to feed.** When they do wake to feed, give them a few minutes before picking them up, espe-cially if they're not fussing too much.

Daytime naps are getting more predictable and may be down to two or three sessions at about the same time every day. Some days will have longer naps than others, and some naps will be skipped altogether. It's more of a routine now, but it's not completely predictable. To help your baby nap better, the single most important step you can take is to put them down before they're really tired and cranky. Don't keep a baby awake, thinking that may tire them out and lead to better sleep; it just doesn't work that way. That's because your baby is still learning how to fall asleep, and at these early stages, they're not very good at it yet. They'll find it easier to succeed in this new skill if they're not too tired and strung out.

MENTAL AND SOCIAL DEVELOPMENT

Between one and two months of age, your baby's social and mental skills really start to blossom. Sure, they were cute when first born, and it's nice to hold and smell little babies. But now, you'll start to enjoy more complex interactions and back-and-forth communication. It's wonderful.

By two months, most babies have developed a genuine social smile. This is more than a random muscle contraction; it's a smile that conveys happiness. You'll see it when they recognize your face, if you make a funny sound, or if the dog licks their foot. You may also see other facial expressions, sometimes copying your mood, like a pout or a gloomy frown. Sharing moods through these expressions is the first step in genuine two-way communication.

There will be more vocalizations and sounds now as your baby starts practicing with their vocal cords. You'll hear the start of "coos" or soft single-vowel sounds like "aaaaah" or "eeeeeh." You might get little screeches or yelps, too. It's all about experimentation and practice.

To help encourage these early communication skills, the most important contribution you can make is to notice and react. Repeat back what they say, or add your own commentary. Say, "Yeah, oooooh, I agree. Mom's perfume smells nice!" React to smiles with your own bigger smile; react to sad faces with your own sad face and a tale of woe: "I know, right? That's the last slice of pizza!" Try to elicit your baby's reactions, and let their noises and faces trigger your own reactions in ways they can see and hear.

Here's a quick way to remember:

- **React (Good!):** Do something when baby does something. They make a noise, you say "You made a noise!"

- **Interact (Better!):** Go back and forth with your baby's reactions and then your reactions. It's like a game of tennis. They make a coo, you say "Yeah sure, aaaah, you like my new shirt I got on today?" Then they make an "Eeeee" noise and a pout, and you make a sad face and say "Yeah, it cost a lot." Then repeat.

- **Overact (Best!):** Sometimes, you have to let it all hang out. Big, exaggerated smiles, overreactions, and silly faces are great ways to have fun and learn together. Turn the dial up to eleven, and ham it up!

HOW TO PLAY

Playtime routines are getting more interactive now, and it's a fun time for learning, too. You may have already come up with some special daddy games to share. Here are a few more ideas:

- **"Get it!":** Use colorful, blocky toys that maybe rattle, and gently move them around for your baby to reach for and swat at. Hand-eye coordination is just starting to emerge. You'll want to help your baby get the hang of this by holding their hand to assist.

- **Moving parts:** Gently bicycle your baby's legs, or move their arms into different positions while explaining what you're doing.

I don't mean to imply that every hour of every day has to be filled with talking and reacting and playing. Your baby can (and should) spend some time on their own (with you nearby but not necessarily *always* engaged). Learning to entertain yourself is another good skill.

OUTINGS WITH YOUR NEWBORN

Almost anywhere you go, you can take your baby. The change of scenery and opportunity to see, hear, and smell new things will be good for both of you. You can go with your partner, too, as a family, or just offer to take baby on an outing. The hardware store, a brewery tour, the coffee shop, a park, the corner with all the pigeons—it's all good. You don't need anyplace especially fancy or expensive to have a good trip.

You'll probably want to start small, since younger babies get tired and cranky quickly. Avoid really loud places until you can provide safe ear protection (no shooting ranges, no monster truck rallies).

Always travel safely, with a vehicle safety seat. You'll probably bring a stroller, and you'll definitely bring a diaper bag. If it's a super hot or sunny day, avoid the heat of midday and try to stay in the shade. You can also use a mineral-based sunscreen (containing zinc oxide or titanium dioxide), along with long sleeves, a big hat, or whatever other gear you need for the weather.

MONTH TWO WELL VISIT AND IMMUNIZATIONS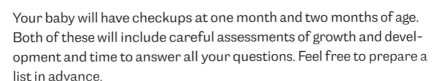

Your baby will have checkups at one month and two months of age. Both of these will include careful assessments of growth and development and time to answer all your questions. Feel free to prepare a list in advance.

The two-month visit also includes a set of vaccines or immunizations. Your baby is vulnerable now to a lot of infections that you haven't had to worry about because your family had you vaccinated and because almost all of us have received these same vaccines. When nearly everyone is vaccinated, it helps protect all of us, including even infants too young to have gotten all their doses yet.

The two-month vaccines are given with combination products so fewer injections are needed. Protection will be built against the following:

- Diphtheria, tetanus (lockjaw), and pertussis (whooping cough)

- HIB and pneumococcus, two bacteria that cause meningitis and blood poisoning

- Hepatitis B

- Polio

- Rotavirus, a virus that can cause severe diarrhea

Most babies have no side effects at all from any of these. Some babies will get a little bit of fever or some fussiness as their immune systems crank up and learn to fight. Your pediatrician will tell you how to use a safe dose of acetaminophen after vaccines if it's necessary. If your baby seems to be having any kind of serious or unexpected reaction after vaccines, contact your pediatrician right away. I've gotten less than a handful of these calls in twenty-five years of practice, but please don't hesitate to call your baby's doctor if you're worried after any vaccines.

PARTNER CHECK-IN

You've got some routines now and a growing sense of confidence. But having a little baby is still a whole lot of work for you and your partner. You may both be feeling the weight of the work and the lack of sleep and might feel there's no end in sight.

Be open and honest with your partner about where you both are mentally. Talk about positive experiences and cute times with your baby but also those times when you've been feeling down. You can be most supportive of each other by sharing and listening.

Your baby's second month is an important time to try to reconnect as a couple. It's been baby-baby-baby now for almost two months. Think about making plans to go out, leaving your baby with grandma or a trusted friend. Even for just a few hours, try to focus on each other, you and your partner. Your baby is important and needs you. And you and your partner need each other, too.

SELF CHECK-IN

Dads need to take care of themselves, too. You've probably returned to your job by now, and you need to try to work in some time for the hobbies and things you used to enjoy. Some of them, like listening to music, you can share with your baby (dance, too!). Some of them, maybe not so much—you can keep blacksmithing or glass blowing just on your own for now.

One thing that can help nearly every new dad: exercise. Good, sweaty exercise at least a couple of times a week can lift your mood and help you sleep better. If you don't have time to get to the gym, go for a run in the neighborhood. Or start a one-hundred push-ups challenge in your basement. You might feel tired and stressed and maybe lazy. If you force yourself to move, you'll feel better afterward.

Reach out to trusted friends and family. Don't be afraid to be vulnerable, and don't hesitate to reach out for comfort and support when you need it. You may never have needed to have mental health conversations before, but it's important to recognize your limits so you don't spin into burnout and depression. Talking about your mood can be challenging or uncomfortable at first. Remember that people in your life want to support you. Give them the chance.

MONTH TWO: MILESTONE CONCERNS

Babies don't all develop the same skills at the same time. But if your baby is still doing these things by the time they're two months of age, you should talk with their pediatrician.

- Eyes are crossing often or most of the time

- Not reacting to loud sounds

- Doesn't move hands toward mouth

- Can't lift head off the floor while lying on stomach, even for a moment

- Stays floppy or weak

- Seems especially stiff

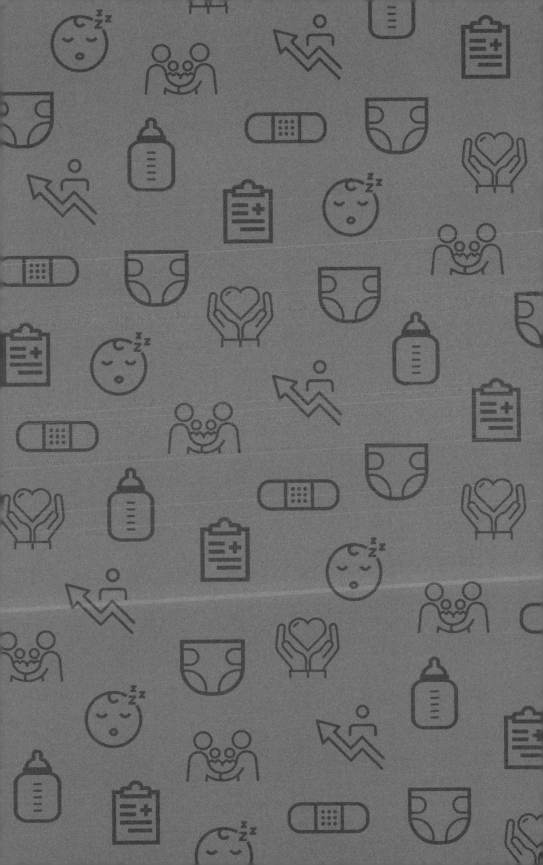

CHAPTER EIGHT

THE THIRD MONTH WITH YOUR NEWBORN

You've made it past most of the newborn fussiness, and sleep is improving. At the same time, your baby is smiling, and you can feel the warmth and the love. The third month is a magical time.

The theme of this third month is growth. Not just physical growth but the blossoming and growth of your baby's own personality and way of looking at the world. You're growing, too, as a dad and a partner. There are challenges and new things for all three of you to learn and new horizons every single day.

In this chapter, we'll cover the growth of your baby's physical and cognitive skills in the third month and how you can help. Sleeping, crying, feeding, pooping—we've got it covered, along with tips on taking care of yourself and your partner. Stop and think about how far you've come and how many surprises and smiles are ahead. Your journey has begun, and the best is yet to come.

GROWTH AND APPEARANCE

In the third month, expect about another one and a half to two pounds of weight gain and growth of an inch or so. It's okay if your baby is growing a little more or a little less. Your baby's own sense of appetite and hunger will work very well at making sure they're getting the right amount to eat. If your baby isn't gaining quite as fast as expected, your pediatrician may suggest altering your feeding style or schedule, but don't worry about this unless your pediatrician wants you to make changes.

Is it possible for a young baby to overeat and become overweight? The short answer is no. Let them eat when they're hungry. However, there are things you can do to avoid falling into habits that can contribute to overeating later. Stop feeding your baby when they're satisfied and done. Don't push them to finish a bottle or stay longer at the breast. Don't offer cereal or any other complementary foods yet. Stay away from juice. And keep in mind that fussing and crying don't always mean your baby is hungry. Maybe they're bored and want some playtime with dad!

MOVEMENT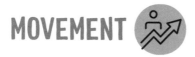

Your baby is becoming stronger, with a vastly improved ability to control and coordinate movements. By the end of this month, they can lift their head up well when lying on their stomach and push up with their arms to support their chest. They want to get up higher so they can see what's going on. When held upright, say while sitting on your hip bone, they'll keep their head up steady and strong.

Hand skills are improving, too. They'll take a swat at objects and might even start to aim correctly once in a while. Though your baby will often bat with a closed fist, they can open their hands to grasp and maybe even shake objects now.

Their lower body and legs are stronger, too. When you hold them upright, they'll extend their legs and try to stand. They probably have the strength to push upward but won't have a great sense of balance yet, so hold tight if they start jumping. Don't worry about putting too much pressure on the legs; if they're having fun and smiling, that means nothing hurts. When your baby is tired of standing, they will let you know.

SENSORY DEVELOPMENT

Your baby's sight has continued to improve and their memory, too! When you walk into a room, they'll see and recognize you from farther away and show excitement with a smile. Your baby will also turn their head toward your "Hey, tiger! Good morning!"

Babies by three months aren't just looking. They're watching closely, studying, and trying to figure out what things are and what they do. They'll stare and get wide-eyed at objects they find especially interesting or exciting. Your baby can now perceive objects separately from their backgrounds, and they're super curious about faces, bright things, moving things, and things that are new or unusual. Moving objects can now be tracked easily with smooth and coordinated eye movements.

Three-month-olds will reach for and bat at objects, though they'll still miss at that first grab sometimes. Help them practice and develop hand-eye skills. It takes time to learn, and your baby will love practicing and improving!

Your baby will have fun exploring touch and other senses, too. Let them stroke and pull your beard or hair and feel a smooth plastic ball, and say words to describe the sensations. Name unusual sounds or smells, too. You might say, "That's an ambulance going by," or "That croaky noise is a frog in the bushes," or "That's mom's morning coffee smell!"

FEEDING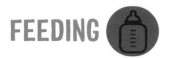

Overall, by the third month, most babies have stretched out the time between feedings. They're often following a fairly predictable schedule. As always, follow those hunger cues. There will be growth spurts and times of both increased and decreased appetite. The only intake needed at this age is breast milk, infant formula, or a combination of both. Infants who are exclusively breastfed should still receive their daily vitamin D supplement.

Nursing babies at three months are feeding about eight times a day, often with longer stretches at night and closer together feedings by day. Formula-fed babies are typically taking about six feeds a day, with about five to six ounces per bottle. More or fewer feedings are fine, too.

Night feeding is still occurring for most babies, but at least by now they'll go back to sleep after a snack. When your baby wakes for a night feed, you can delay starting the feed for a few minutes, especially if they're not too upset. Sometimes your baby will go back to sleep without a meal.

In the United States, about half of babies are exclusively breastfed at three months. Many families who had started out breast only have started adding some formula feedings by now. Whatever amount, if any, of breastfeeding or pumping that your partner is doing is fine. It can be especially difficult to keep up with nursing if your partner must return to work. Be supportive either way. The best way of feeding your baby can include breast, bottles, and formula. A fed, happy, and healthy mom and baby is the goal.

Helpful neighbors and family may suggest starting cereal soon, perhaps by adding it to your baby's formula in a bottle. This is not a good idea. Early cereal does not help sleep. Your baby doesn't need added food yet. That will come later.

MONTH THREE: HEALTHY POOP

Here's something you probably haven't thought about: What makes poop stink? It's bacteria! By now, your baby's gut has become colonized with healthy bacteria to aid digestion, and you'll smell it in the poop. Odor can also change with diet (breastfed babies may have a "sweeter" smell) and how long the food has been digesting (less frequent stools are more pungent). Your three-month-old may have an almost adult-looking and smelling poop by now, with a more formed consistency and a brownish color. Don't worry if there are some changes day to day in stool color, smell, or consistency. Your baby's gut and bacteria are still changing, developing, and maturing.

COLIC AND CRYING

Your baby still cries some. Thankfully, they've got other ways to communicate now, and the daily amount of crying has trailed off. There'll be fewer crying episodes, and it's become easier to console crying. Still, there will be times when you'll be back to using tried-and-true soothing methods, like holding and rocking. Look for newer ways to distract, too, like singing a song, tickling, or blowing raspberries. You know your baby. Do what works!

If your baby is crying for more than an hour a day or has an abrupt increase or change in a crying pattern, visit their doctor.

SLEEPING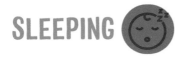

Sleep patterns change dramatically by the end of the third month. By now, your baby is sleeping for about fifteen out of every twenty-four hours, more or less, with a larger percentage of sleep at night. Though most babies won't quite sleep all the way through, many will sleep at least five to six hours in a row, get up to eat, and then go back to sleep.

Most babies are taking two or maybe three naps a day at about the same time each day. These are followed by longer times of awake and playtime.

Some babies are temperamentally born good sleepers; some fight sleep at every turn; most are in-between. If you've got a super good sleeper, you're lucky. To some degree, sleep quality will also depend on how hard you and your partner push the sleep training. As a general rule, firmer and harder sleep training works quickest but will involve more crying and fussing. Only you and your partner can decide how important sleep is to you and how hard you want to push.

Adapt the three-month sleep tips below to your and your partner's style and goals:

Try to stick to the sleep-eat-play cycle. That is, feed your baby as soon as they wake up rather than feeding them right before the next nap or at bedtime. Separate feeding from falling asleep. In the long run, that's a key step to getting babies to fall asleep and stay asleep on their own.

Put your baby down while they're a little groggy. At naptime and bedtime, you may be tempted to hold them until they are asleep, then quietly put them down. That might seem to work at first, but this will soon backfire. Sneaking away after putting your sleeping baby down will cause more night awakenings. They need to learn to fall asleep all on their own, not relying on your presence. You don't have to do this all at once, but aim to at least try sometimes.

Be consistent with timing, pre-sleep routines, and the sleep setting.

When your baby wakes at night, don't rush to feed. Let them fuss a few minutes and even longer if they're not hysterical. They won't learn to fall back asleep on their own if you never give them a chance.

MENTAL AND SOCIAL DEVELOPMENT

Your baby will smile back at strangers, but they know who you are and will save the biggest smiles for their parents. They know you by sight, by the sound of your voice, and probably by your scent, too. They may even recognize the sound of your car coming home and get excited before you reach the door.

With their rapidly growing brain and intellect, the world has become a fascinating place for your baby, filled with wonderful new things. You'll see your baby's interest in things like a bird's chirp, the spinning plate in the microwave, or their own adorable toes. Many babies have started to giggle or laugh out loud by now. Here's a good way to get a belly laugh: Nibble on the side of their chest or back, make "nom nom nom" noises, and say "Mmmmm! Delicious baby!"

Your baby loves watching you but wants more interaction and back-and-forth games now, like peekaboo or swatting at toys or balloons. They might even pout or cry when a game ends. That's not a sign that they're spoiled. It means they have a healthy attachment and are trying to express how they feel.

Vocal skills have improved, too, with more elaborate cooing and the start of babbling with consonant sounds. Sometimes raspberries and spit bubbles, too! They're all forms of vocalizations. Your baby won't be talking or making sense literally yet, but start to get in the habit of answering anyway. Let the conversation volley back and forth so they can practice how talking with someone works:

You: "Good holding call there."

Baby: "Gaaaaaaa."

You: "Yeah, you're right. That gives us a first down."

Baby: spits and blows a raspberry

You: "Seriously? You want a quarterback sneak now?"

If you have a bilingual household, I strongly encourage you and your partner to speak in both languages. Your baby, with their amazing developing brain, can learn two (or more) languages at the same time.

Building trusting and reciprocal relationships should include other people, too. Your baby should spend some time being held by and playing with other adults—family, friends, whomever you hang out with. Everyone will have a little different play style and a different way of interacting, and that's great.

HOW TO PLAY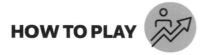

You've already found games your baby likes (see pages 81 and 94). Feel free to adapt and make games a little more complicated as they grow. Here are some new ideas that work great for three-month-olds:

Race car: Hold baby in your lap, facing away, and hold their hands like they're on a steering wheel. Countdown three, two, one, and the race is on! Steer right! Steer left! Avoid the cow!

Sing-along: Classic baby sing-alongs have surprise endings ("Pop! goes the weasel!") or hand motions (my own dad never got the itsy-bitsy spider movements right with his grandkids, but they loved it anyway).

Reading: It is never too early. Pick books with big colorful pictures and pages to grab and manipulate. Talk and point to things on each page. Add sound effects and special voices. Own it!

TRAVELING WITH YOUR NEWBORN

Around the three-month mark, traveling with your baby gets a lot easier. You've got routines settled and better sleep, and they're perky and happy and eager to meet people. You might want to start small with a shorter and closer trip or go crazy and head across the country or to a resort in Mexico. (You may need a passport, even for a newborn. Check first.) Here are a few specific tips:

Car trips: Safety is crucial. Your baby should always travel in a secure safety seat. Plan frequent stops for feeding and unwinding. Though you don't want to routinely have your baby sleep at home in a car seat on an incline, if your baby falls asleep on a long trip, it's okay to keep going. Use a mirror or video camera to keep an eye on them, or mom or dad can sit in the back.

Planes: Unless it's a short ride, you'll want to pay extra for your baby to get their own seat so you have somewhere to strap in the safety seat. Alternatively, you can hold your baby and check the car seat to your destination. Some babies have ear pain from pressure changes during ascent and descent. Avoid this by having your baby take a bottle or nurse at these times.

Trains: It's hard to beat the comfort and safety of a train. You and your partner can stretch out and take turns holding and playing. Big windows offer a lot to look at, too.

Consider traveling during your child's usual sleep time, and bring backup clothes, diapers, and other supplies, more than you think you'll need. Delays or traffic may mess with your careful plans.

PARTNER CHECK-IN

The third month can be a time of joy and, finally, some relaxation. Newborn fussiness has improved, and there are big smiles now and a baby who is starting to truly enjoy being alive. Your partner may feel energized and ready for new challenges.

Or maybe not. Some moms feel exhausted and strung out, especially if they're back to work full-time. They may be realizing that the work of being a mom isn't what they had pictured. Their bodies still aren't cooperating, and they're just not feeling like themselves.

Be honest and open with your partner and ready to listen to what she says and how she's saying it. Don't assume she feels the way you do or that because she isn't complaining she hasn't got much on her mind. Ask her. Find quiet time to talk and listen. Resist the urge to try to "fix" things and offer unsolicited advice. Start by listening, truly listening, and think about what her fundamental needs are and how you can support them.

Do this at a time when one of you isn't holding your baby, either. If you haven't done it yet, make concrete plans to get out as a couple, using family or friends as a sitter, if only for a few hours. Many hotels offer day use rates that are a fraction of the cost of an overnight stay. This can give you an oasis for some intimacy or even just a spot to take a long, uninterrupted shower and a solid nap. Remember that the health and happiness of your baby depends on the health and happiness of you two parents and your partnership together.

Symptoms of postpartum mental illness, including depression and anxiety, can begin or peak anytime in the first year of life. If you're feeling that your partner is in an especially low place and you don't know how to help, contact her physician. The U.S. National Mental Health Suicide and Crisis Lifeline is 988. Dial that from any phone, anytime.

About sex: The standard advice is that women, after birth or C-section, should abstain from sex for six weeks. That's a reasonable generalization, but that's all it is. Your partner may or may not feel physically or mentally ready for sex on an exact schedule. She's tired and doesn't feel like herself. Remind her that you love her, be patient, and talk about your feelings without the pressure of expectations. Take it slow. When the time is right, remember the lube.

SELF CHECK-IN

How is your overall mental health and well-being? Are you sleeping okay and eating reasonably well? Getting a little exercise? Have you got the mental energy to get your home and work jobs done? If not, it may be time for you to speak with your physician, a mental health professional, or a trusted friend or mentor. Don't be scared or ashamed to ask for help.

Be wary of falling into a comparison trap. You may know another baby that's sleeping better or is wearing bigger clothes or who seems to have reached some milestones quicker. Or you may have a neighbor whose partner seems more energetic. You might feel a little defeated or jealous. Instead, try to focus on all the great things your baby is learning to do and all the progress you've made as a family.

Now is also a good time to ask yourself: Am I becoming the dad I want to be and the dad that reflects who I really am? There are lots of great ways to be a dad. You'll at times be silly or serious or affectionate. There are times when you'll concentrate on being a provider or a responsible parent guiding your child on a straight and narrow path. Or you may see yourself as more of a nurturing dad, helping your child find their own way with your encouragement rather than guidance. None of these are the best way or the only way. Figure out which is your way.

If you're not the dad you want to be, ask yourself why. Think about what you can do to be a different dad. Give yourself some slack to make mistakes and change course. Being a dad has become what you are, but it's not all that you are. To be the best dad, you have to be yourself. It's normal to have times when you feel down, but you should be enjoying yourself, too. You should be having fun with your baby and your partner, maybe not all the time but often enough to feel that you're on the right path.

MONTH THREE: MILESTONE CONCERNS

Although babies grow and develop at different rates, there are some things we expect almost all three-month-old babies to do. If your baby isn't meeting some or all of these steps, talk with your pediatrician:

- Isn't responding to noises

- Isn't watching things move with their eyes

- Doesn't grasp, hold, or try to reach for objects or toys

- Doesn't pay attention to new faces

- Doesn't calm down when you pick them up, at least for a little while

- Has arms or legs that are floppy or rarely move or has movements that are becoming less brisk and coordinated

- Has one body side that's stronger or stiffer than the other

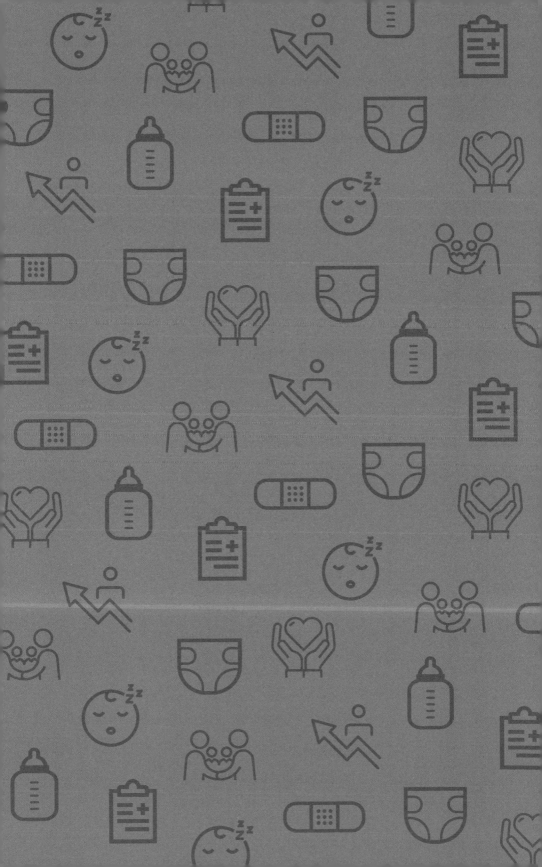

LOOKING AHEAD

Congrats, you've made it through the first three months! Think about how much has changed, in expected and unexpected ways. You knew you'd be having a baby, but did you think about just how special holding them could be? Your tiny newborn has grown into a smiling baby with their own personality and their own way of looking at the world. Do they make faces like you, or do they remind you of their mom? The first time they nursed or took a bottle might seem like ages ago now. You've become a full-time, full-fledged, and certified dad.

You and your baby have a whole lot more to look forward to. They'll start a variety of complementary foods between four and six months, and you'll probably sneak in a taste of your ice cream or a cookie. Babies can usually sit up completely on their own by seven months, freeing up their hands for manipulative play and learning to clap or make the "touchdown!" gesture. There will be some stranger anxiety, starting by nine months, and you'll be there to reassure them and help them understand that Uncle Lee isn't such a weirdo after all. You'll read new books together, sing silly made-up songs, and go on dozens of trips and journeys. Every grocery run or trip to pick up tacos can be an adventure!

Around twelve months, most babies say their first words. It might be the name of their favorite guy in the world: "Dad." Or they might call you "Dada" or "Daaaa." Or, honestly, the first word might be the name of your dog. Who knows? It will be adorable either way.

Your journey with your child has only just begun. You've got lots of memories to make and lots of lessons to teach. You'll both make a few mistakes, and you'll both grow and learn. And you'll do it together.

INDEX

Diaper changes, 22–23, 41–42
Diaper rash cream, 23, 41
Diapers, 22, 41
Diphtheria, tetanus, and pertussis
    vaccine, 96
Dressing baby, 39

E

Emotional self-care, 63–64, 85, 97, 111
Eye drops, 33
Eyes, watery/gunky, 83

F

Failure to progress, 11
Family
  as childcare providers, 19
  communicating with, 5–6
Family and Medical Leave Act
    (FMLA), 76
Feeding
  after sleep, 80, 106
  breastfeeding, 44–45, 68, 104
  burping baby, 47
  cluster, 46–47
  first feedings, 32
  first month, 77–78
  formula, 45–46, 68, 77–78, 90
  gas, 47, 78, 90
  healthy habits, 102
  hiccups, 47
  night, 70, 77, 90, 92, 104, 106
  second month, 89–90
  spit-up, 47, 77
  supplies, 25–26
  third month, 104
  week one, 67–68
First aid kits, 26
First month. *See* Month one
First words, 114
Formula feeding, 45–46, 68, 90
Free-range parenting, 7
Friends
  as childcare providers, 19
  communicating with, 5–6

G

Gas, 47, 78, 90
Gentle parenting, 7
Gliders, 26
Growth
  first month, 74

second month, 88
  third month, 102
Grunting baby syndrome, 49

H

Health challenges, 11–13
Heart murmurs, 11
Hepatitis B vaccine, 34, 96
Hiccups, 47
Holding baby, 38–39
Hospital, leaving after birth, 60

I

Immunizations, 34, 95–96
Inclined sleepers, avoiding, 22
Infant dyschezia, 49
Injuries, birth, 11–12
Instinctive parenting, 7

J

Jaundice, 11, 35

L

Lactation specialists, 44–45
Laundry, 23, 27

M

Mattresses, 21–22
Measurements, post-birth, 32–33
Meconium, 48
Mental development
  first month, 80–81
  second month, 93–95
  third month, 107–108
Mental health
  dad's, 63–64, 85
  partner's, 13, 62–63, 84
Midwives, questions to ask, 9
Milestones
  first month concerns, 83
  premature babies, 11
  second month concerns, 98
  third month concerns, 112
  use of term, 54
  week one, 64–65
Milk supply, increasing, 45
Money-saving tips, 27
Month one
  feeding, 77–78
  growth and appearance, 74

ABOUT THE AUTHOR

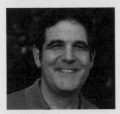 **Roy Benaroch** is a general pediatrician and adjunct professor of pediatrics at Emory University. He's created hundreds of hours of educational and entertaining audio and video material for parents and medical professionals. This is his fourth book for parents. He and his wife have raised three children and live with their two Yorkshire terriers near Atlanta, Georgia.